The Art of Self - Defense

(A do-it-yourself, Self-defense guide for security personnel & for the layman)

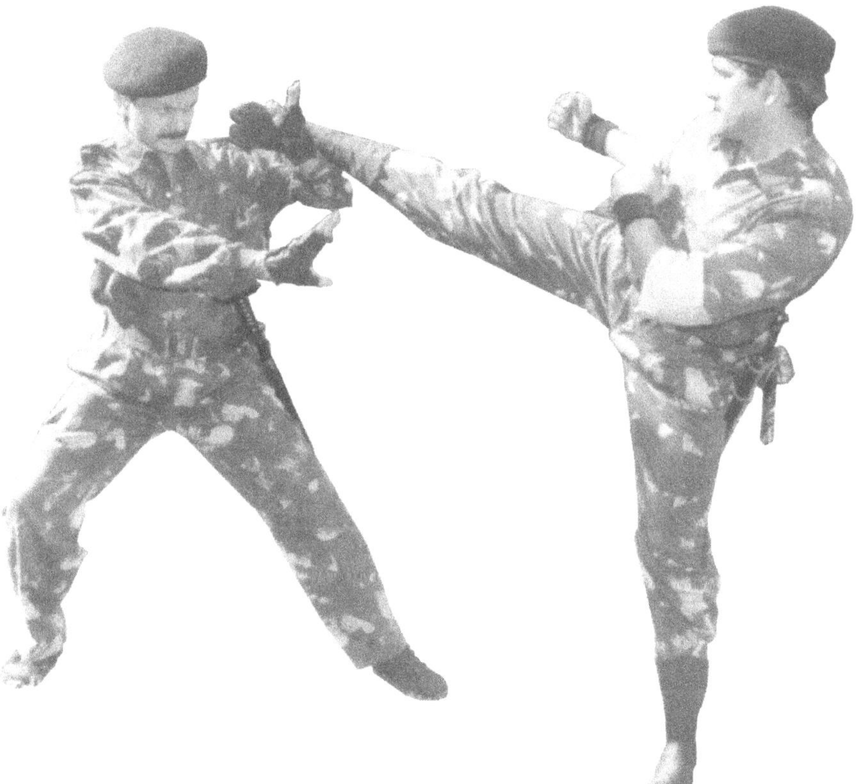

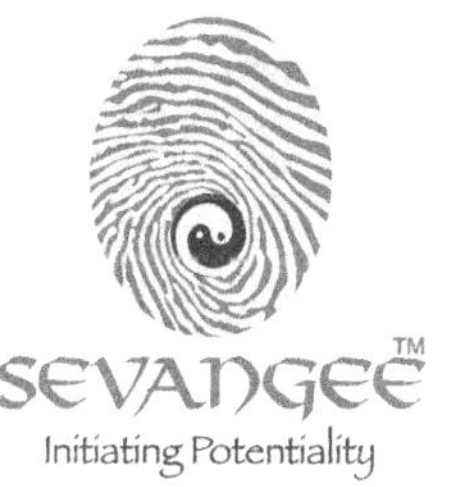

Christopher Fernandes
& Lazarus Mascarenhas

SEVANGEE
Initiating Potentiality

The Art of Self Defense
(A do-it-yourself, self-defense guide for security personnel and for the lay-man)
By *Christopher Fernandes & Lazarus Mascarenhas*

Printed in India.

Published and Distributed by:

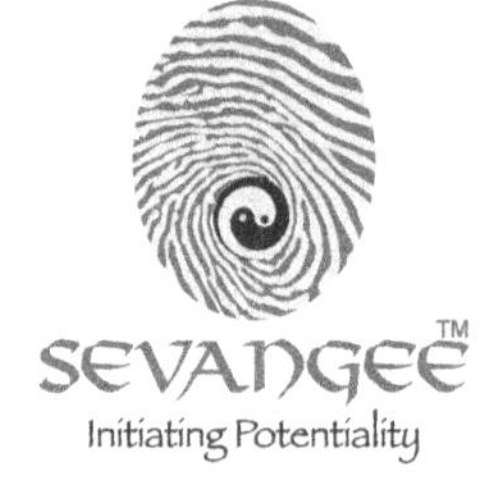

Sevangee Publications
73, Sher-e-Punjab,
Andheri (East),
Mumbai 400 093,
India.
Website: www.sevangee.com
Email: info@sevangee.com

Second Edition (2019): ISBN No: 978-81-934689-0-6

This manual is dedicated to a very special group of people who often go unnoticed and unrewarded in their dedication and commitment to preserving life and enhancing the security of others.

.....to the personnel of the armed forces – the army, navy, air force, and paramilitary forces, who go through rigorous years of training, face the vagaries of unfamiliar terrain and risk their lives in the defense of the nation.

.....to the police force who work long and strenuous hours of duty, and also risk their lives in maintaining law and order within the country.

.....and to all similar professionals, body guards and security professional who thro their profession ensure the safety of others lives even at the risk of their own.

May the secrets techniques of the martial arts spelt out in this book, enhance their capabilities and reduce the risk to their lives in their commitment to the defense of others and security.

Just by reading a book on swimming you cannot become a swimmer, so also in the same way with self defense. In this field it is 90% practice and 10% knowledge. A practitioner must start at the beginning and proceed to the next lesson only when he has mastered the first lesson. This book has been laid out with that purpose in mind and it would be defeating its purpose to open it to a later section and try to master the techniques there without first learning the basics.

1. Practice each steps slowly, moving from one technique to another, with attention towards technical excellence.

2. When your movements become fluid you may increase your speed without discomfort or loss of control so that the technique becomes instinctive.

3. Do not be hesitant to repeat the technique even after you have moved on to a subsequent technique. 'Slow and steady wins the race', is an old proverb, so let's hope for the best.

BEST OF LUCK!

Acknowledgements

We wish to express our sincere appreciation to our students and instructors from Universal Martial Arts Research Centre for their willingness to pose for the photographs. Our sincere thanks to Mr.Upen and Mr.Alexander Fernandes for their excellent photography and the excellent sketches. We would like to thanks Mr. G. Rodrigues for his proof readings. We would also like to thank the late Mr. G.S. Sethi from English Edition for encouraging us to come out with this manual. Our sincere thanks to Mr. Charanjit Singh Gidda for putting the layout for second edition as a E-book. Our sincere thanks to Rev. Fr. Francis Swami s.j. the Principal of Holy Family High School, Andheri (E), who encouraged us and allowed to trained and teach in the school premises and allowed to shoot the photographs in the school premises. Our sincere thanks to Mr. Joseph D'souza who worked silently behind the scene and saw to it the project was completed. We would also like to thank our students, Mr. Mr. Joe D'souza, Mr. Carlton Hill, Mr. Rakesh Menon and Mr. Ravindra Vishwakarma, who willing participated in the photo-shoot. Last but not the least we would like to thanks our wives and children who had been a constant support, for without their encouragement we wouldn't been able to accomplish and achieve this goal.

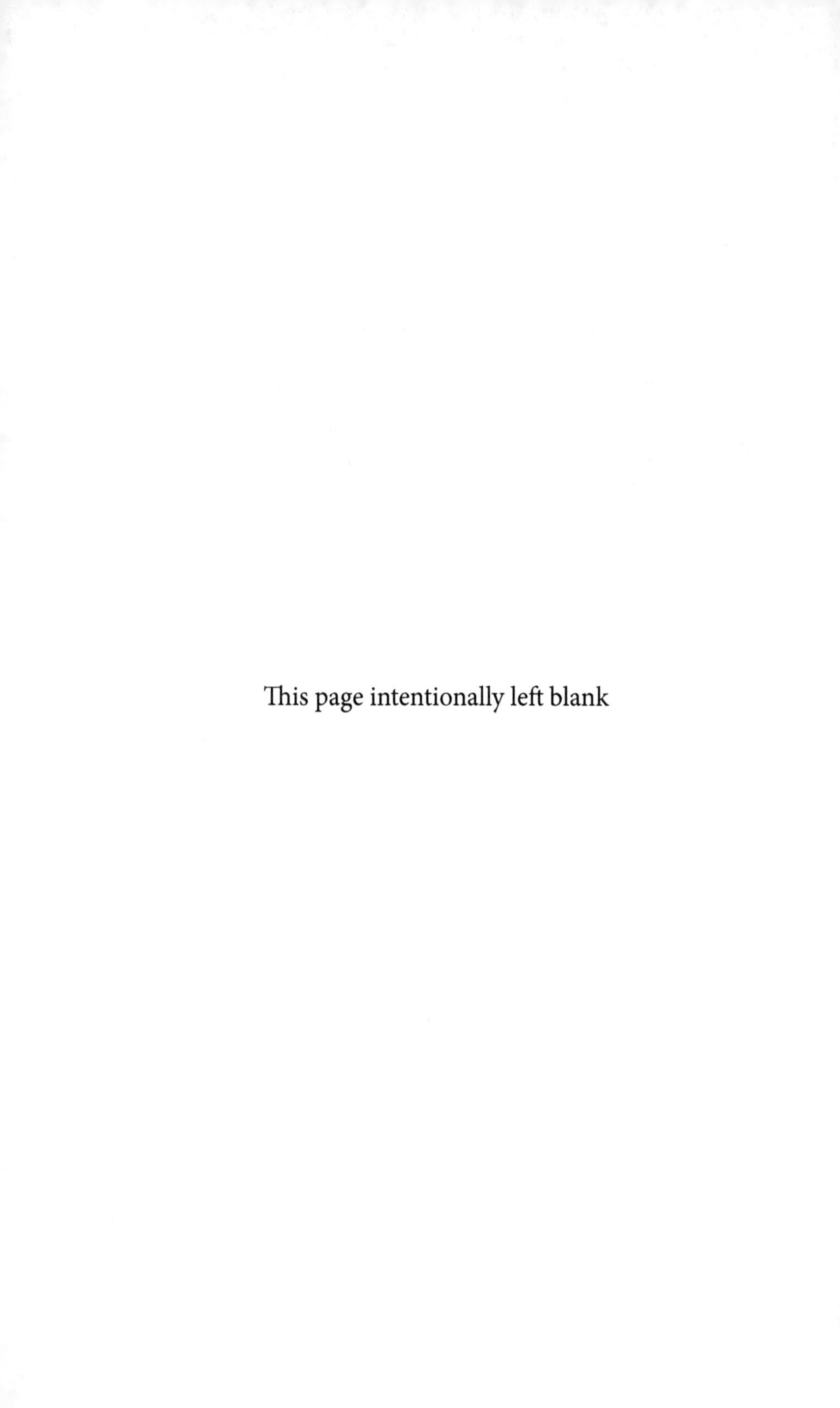

This page intentionally left blank

Contents

This page intentionally left blank

Foreword

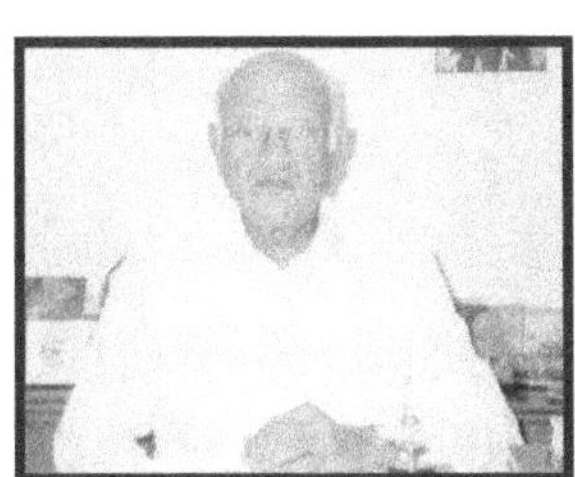

In writing the foreword to, and endorsing this book, I in no way claim to be an expert in the martial arts. However, my years of experience in the Police Force have led me to strongly believe that every citizen should be adequately equipped to defend oneself in an environment of increasing crime.

In the past few decades, there has been a phenomenal increase in crime and consequently the need for protection. Citizens have been licensed to have personal pistols that are expensive, or provided with police protection, which again is costly and a burden on the police force or private security agencies. The propagating of the martial arts while equipping people to protect themselves substitutes "fire-arms" with the strength of the arms, legs, feet,….. the entire body. From firearms that can be destructive and fatal, the martial arts without necessary being fatal, can equip an individual with adequate security through self defense that is effective and controlled.

Self defense through the martial arts will not only make individuals more secure and society safer but lessen the burden and tasks of the police. Training in the martial arts will also contribute to the general health and well being of its adherents. The martial arts a collective accumulation of the experience and insights of centuries and in-depth study of the human body and its strong and weak points have gone into the creation of a scientific system of self defense.

In ancient times it was not unusual for a student to trudge over a thousand miles, scaling high mountains and crossing huge rivers and traveling through dangerous forests to seek the teaching of the great master. It was common practice that subtle techniques, unique experiences and special knowledge were made esoteric and only handed down from father to son and master to selected disciple. Today, even though travel is simplified to eliminate its hardships its still not easy to come across a good teacher who has the knowledge and is willing to hand his secrets over to anyone who knocks at his door.

"The Art of Self-Defense" by Christopher Fernandes and Lazarus Mascarenhas is a book that incorporates a life time of the practice of the martial arts. It's not only their individual experience but also the experience of the masters they have learnt from. It is a book with detailed instructions that with the help of photographs illustrates how each movement can be made effective as a defensive or offensive move if executed correctly. I believe after reading it, you will conclude that this book is like a lighthouse for the ships at sea, or like a signpost along the road for cars on land. I am sure this book will be of great value to the general public, and certainly to the security personnel it will be more of a reference book in the line of duty.

It is my great pleasure to write the foreword to this book.

J.F. RIBEIRO
Ex. Director General of Police.

This page intentionally left blank

Introduction

It is far better to learn one method of Self Defense thoroughly, than it is to learn a little about several methods.

Introduction

Violent encounters aren't something that we like to think about, but they happen every day to regular people just like you, who are totally unprepared to deal with such a life changing situation.

WHAT IS SELF-DEFENSE? It is a set of awareness, assertiveness, and verbal confrontation skills with safety strategies and physical techniques that enable someone to successfully escape resist and survive violent attacks! A good self-defense technique should be psychological awareness and verbal skills, not just physical training.

DOES SELF-DEFENSE WORK? Yes. Self-defense training can increase your options and help you prepare responses to slow down, de-escalate, or interrupt an attack. Like any tool, the more you know about it, the more informed you are to make a decision and use it.

Self-Defense is a serious subject that not many people think about and that even fewer people actually do anything about. We feel that not only does the history of society from the beginning of time reek of violence, but that current society continues as a violent place to live. We can't convince a person of the need for self-defense because we feel it is so self-evident we would be wasting our "proverbial breath" on the subject. What's possibly even more amazing is that insurance is only good while you keep paying. No matter how much insurance you have spent last month, last year, your whole lifetime, once you stop paying, none of that insurance you have paid so much money for does anything for you at all. It is gone. Admittedly self defense training is a form of insurance. Hopefully you would never have to use it. The difference is that once you take up self defense, it is something that you can carry with you and rely upon until the day you die.

Have you ever thought about what you would do if a criminal?
- Broke into your home or hotel room while you were there?
- Tried to kidnap you or your children?
- Tried to rob you as you are walking across a parking lot to your car?
- Tried to rape you?
- Lost his temper and directed his anger at you?
- Began an immediate violent attack on you?

Where Do You Fit In With Violent Encounters? It is interesting to note that the type self defense training taught during times of peace is, as a whole, different than the type of training taught during times of war. The following concept is important to truly understand. In peacetime the only reason you choose to fight is because:

- You are involved in some sporting system where you actually participate in the "ring" by choice i.e. boxing, wrestling, judo, karate, aikido, and ninja, kick-boxing, stick-fighting, etc.

- Or because you are challenged to fight by someone on the street, in some establishment, or anywhere else, and you actually agree to the challenge.

If you don't agree to fight, be assaulted, etc., then you are in the same position as on a battlefield in wartime, no difference. As such, the skills you learn should be the same that you would use on a battlefield as those that you would use in an ornament shop during non-war (peace) time.

It doesn't matter how fun-loving you are. It doesn't matter that you don't want to "fight". Why do you think the term Victim exists? If you agreed to a fight, if you agreed to be robbed, if you agreed to be raped, if you agreed to be kidnapped, if you agreed to be mugged, then you wouldn't be a victim. You would be a willing participant.

Do you think victims got up in the morning and said "Today I will be a victim"? Do you think they knew the time and place they would be a victim? Do you think that only certain people are attacked by others? Do you think that because you have no interest in "fighting" or any other such violent activities that you will be okay? Do you think that a criminal asks a person, "Hi, I wanted to commit some act of violence or crime against you, and are you interested in participating?" Do you think a violent aggressor only attacks people who he feels are his physical contemporaries? Do you think he goes after those stronger or weaker than himself? Do you think he plays fair, such as not using a weapon?

- At any time, any place, anywhere, you could be in the wrong place at the wrong time. A person may be nuts, on drugs, a violent jerk looking for trouble, etc. and you just may happen to be in his presence when he decides to get nasty.
- Or you just may be the person who happens to be the one in the presence of a criminal or multiple criminals who are looking for anyone of any race, creed, color, sex, age, etc. to commit a crime upon.

Just because you are an easy going, peaceful person doesn't make you safe. As a matter of fact, unfortunately, you are a prime piece of meat for a criminal. If you don't care to learn how to defend yourself that is fine. Just don't deceive yourself mentally and say "I never have to worry because I am not interested in violence". It appears that there is a psychology among many people that if they think about self-defense or spend time training in it, that then somehow they are bringing it to them. And that by being totally vulnerable, and saying "I hate violence, I am never going to engage in it" that somehow they will be spared from the targeting sites of criminals. Get this in your head. Violence can happen to anyone, anywhere, any time, with no warning, no provocation, and no interest on your part of being a participant in a violent encounter.

The techniques necessary to render an attacker unconscious are only the most brutal man stopping techniques that either stop his breathing or inflict overload to the central nervous system causing him to be unable to attack. Even though the student may be told that if under real attack, to go for the things that have the highest probability of stopping effect, his trained and practiced reactions are all contrary to this and it has been stated by many instructors throughout the ages that you will do in combat as you do in practice.

- You need to practice the way you would perform in an actual violent attack.

- Holds, grips, and other passive techniques cannot be relied upon in a violent encounter. This includes "pain compliance" techniques, which make you more vulnerable to the attacker, especially if there are multiple assailants as these techniques can only be employed on a single assailant at a time.

- Breaking boards is a fine endeavor requiring concentration, striking power, and focus, but boards don't hit back and boards remain completely still. Hitting a live flesh attacker is completely different. Remember, you won't be attacked by a board.

Today's ever-changing international and national political climates require soldiers and the police force to operate in unstable situations without resorting to deadly force. Soldiers/police force relies on their skills to succeed during crises, requiring them to continually train during times of peace. Combative training is very important for soldiers/police force, there are times in missions when rules of engagement are very specific and (soldiers/police force) need options other than lethal force. Even in peacetime, violence can and does happen; many situations blur the lines of who is friendly and who is foe. By giving these guys another option, it instills confidence that they can handle just about any situation that comes up. The best thing about this is it's not perishable; it's applicable in many situations because of the psychological aspect. They understand better how the mind works, and it helps to relate to other soldiers, team members and those whom you're forced to defend yourself against.

❑ ❑ ❑

Chapter 1

Pros & Cons of Self Defense

The goal of Self Defense is not to win a fight, but to escape from an opponent without getting hurt.

Pros & Cons of Self Defense

Combat training teaches us, how to effectively use the body's natural weapons. It is imperative to learn how to properly use your body and its natural weapons to their maximum potential. It is more than just learning specific techniques; it is how to get the most out of them with your body. Learn how to counter the most common and dangerous types of criminal assaults. Ability in self defense can also have an effect on a person's personality. When you are not physically afraid of other people you are more likely to stick up for your rights and assert yourself where you should. In other words, the ability will make you more self confident. In turn, potential troublemakers will avoid you when they sense your self-confidence. Knowing some of the possible causes of violence may help in avoiding it.

Learn how to train effectively when the stakes are life or death:

Training in full contact sparring will not do it, as a matter of fact; it will inculcate all of the incorrect reactions necessary for a real life violent encounter. You are not winning a match; you are saving your life. If you walk off the mat and no one is crippled or maimed, how effective can this approach be? The sporting mindset is not the combative mindset no matter how brutal "The Match". Adapting your mind to a very violent situation and as well as to a difficult situations in general, is a very critical aspect of training. Being aware and recognizing the criminal setups and implementing the procedures that prevent you from being a target is very important.

Learn to understand the element of Fear:

Cultivate your personal "radar" for heightened awareness. Learn, practice and be efficient in execution of the techniques, till it become in second nature. With practice your maneuvers can be made to look quite natural and not the actions of someone suffering from a persecution complex. You don't have to be a black belt expert to defend yourself. Learn how to stand and position yourself in every day life (see Appendix II). Cultivate the element of surprise; anyone can be defeated with the element of surprise. This is of such grave importance that every student must always contemplate its use. This can nullify age difference, strength, size, ability, and skill. Utilize the bodies natural stress response for a counter attack beyond anything you imagined you can do. The response sometimes called "Fear" is never to be eliminated in ones mindset. It can't be eliminated and you wouldn't want it to be anyway.

Learn the myths and realities of self-defense in general:

There is no "magic shield" body position of defense or a magic "one stop shot" when the attack is real. Gain more confidence than you've ever had before. You will experience why the development of self-defense ability increases self-esteem and confidence, and its application to other areas or aspects of an individual's life. Maximize your training time with only the necessary element. It's better to practice 10 minutes a day than 2 hours twice a week. This manual will cultivate physical conditioning, technique mastery, and mental conditioning. Learning how to use any object at hand to significantly increase your ability to defeat your attackers, when the "use of force" is legally justified: like using Pressure Point.

What are your self-defense options?

1. DO NOTHING: You can do nothing at all to be prepared for an assault against you. Maybe it never will happen anyway. Hopefully it won't. The only problem with this strategy is that if it ever does happen, you will be a perfect victim.

2. HIRE A BODYGUARD: How practical is that for most people? And even if you have one(s), are they with you every where you go? With this book you will become your own bodyguard by learning the skills yourself, that can save your own life. Unfortunately, if you are ever in a situation requiring self-defense or personal protection, you are going to be either the victim or victor, but there is a high degree of probability, that no one is going to be there to take care of the problem for you. Relying on strangers near you to risk their lives to protect you is a pretty shaky thing to rely on. Not to mention the fact that even if a willing stranger has the heart to get involved to help you, it doesn't mean that he has the skill and ability to protect you even if he has the heart.

3. POLICE: The police are the closest thing to a government provided bodyguard but, they aren't assigned to follow you around and protect you as an individual, which is what a bodyguard does. They are there to maintain the order of the collective of society which does include you as an individual as part of the whole. If they happen to be right next to you, the chances are low that a criminal or just plain violent jerk is going to decide to attack you in the presence of a police officer. So even with the "best police force", they aren't there with you. It's simply a matter of physics. You get attacked, someone has to see it, report it, and the police have to get there. Now assuming people see it, immediately report it, the dispatch system works perfectly, and there is an officer(s) available to immediately respond, your self-defense situation will most likely be over by then, either way it turns out. Also contrary to the ignorant beliefs of the public, police by law are not required to risk their lives to save yours. This is a simple fact. What this means is that if an attacker is attacking you with a knife, baseball bat or just their bare hands for example, by law, a police officer is not required to jump in-between and risk their life for you like the films. And if you and the attacker are close together, shooting the attacker could be problematic for the officer as he or she may have a hard time hitting the right target. The officer may jump in and save the day. But it is by choice, not job description. Also this is by no means saying that there aren't many fine police officers who put their lives on the line saving people every day. It is just a common trait among criminals that they generally don't like to attack a person in the presence of police officers. And that you can't 100% rely on the fact that any person, including a law enforcement official, will immediately intervene on your behalf with a high risk of personal injury or death to him or herself.

4. GUN: You can carry a gun. A few issues to think about are, although totally in conflict with your constitutional rights, in many states it is illegal to carry a gun. A gun not at your disposal when in need is less helpful than a cup of tea in your hand, literally speaking. If you get a permit and are able to legally carry a gun:

1. it still isn't legal to take with you everywhere such as on an airplane, etc., but

2. more importantly, why do you think the masters of combat in WW II developed a system of vicious hand-to-hand combat since the legality of a soldier carrying a gun was no moot point.

As a matter of fact, carrying a machine gun, grenade launcher, flame-thrower, big combat knife, mini steel shovel etc. were all part of a soldiers repertoire. Now let's get out of wartime. Let's go to "peacetime". The rules are even harder. In war, a soldier doesn't have to worry about drawing a weapon, it is drawn always. The soldier doesn't have to worry about shooting the enemy, which is someone threatening him. But now we're a civilian in peacetime. The bottom line is that even if you have a gun on your person, just draw it on any suspecting or threatening person that comes up to you and see how fast you end up in jail. Or don't draw it until you are attacked and see how useful it is to try to draw a weapon when your person is suddenly attacked. Good luck on making it through the encounter. That's why speed drawing can be a dangerous focus to train on and rely upon. While you're trying to draw your weapon, your assailant is taking you apart. Draw or Don't Draw is a nice Catch 22 situation made much worse by our wonderfully evolving legal system.

5. OTHER WEAPONS: Aside from the gun issue then, perhaps you carry a crowbar, bat, club, machete, collapsible baton, etc. in your car. Well, first you could still have legal problems depending upon what an officer feels is right or wrong about either the "weapon" or why the thing, such as a crowbar, is in the front seat or under the seat. Secondly, do you know how to use it? You could be really hurt by someone grabbing what you think is a weapon, and you don't know how to use it, and then your assailant isn't intimidated at all by it, and then you are in deadly trouble. Without any proper combat training, you don't have the mindset or skill to be fooling around with such things. Thirdly, again are you going to carry a crowbar with you into the grocery store and everywhere else? A weapon not at your disposal when in need is less helpful than a cup of tea in your hand, literally speaking.

6. KNIFE: How about a knife. While still not legal in many areas, it is less illegal to carry in most places than a gun. It is small enough to carry with you concealed or unconcealed. But again you have the same problems as with a gun and sometimes even worse. You have the Draw / Don't Draw issue. Draw a knife on someone who may be a threat and you have a good chance of ending up in jail. Don't draw and have fun getting to it while you are suddenly attacked. Stabbings are messy and no one, especially cops, likes the site of knife wounds. That means a higher probability of a "go straight to jail" card. And just like with other weapons, without knife training, which is an extension of hand to hand combat training, you sure as hell better be able to take down your assailant or he may take it away from you and use it on you and again, you aren't trained to fight an unarmed assailant hand to hand without a knife, so you are really in deep trouble if he has a knife.

7. PEPPER SPRAY/STUN GUNS (Non-Lethal): If you are worried about hurting a scumbag who wants to hurt you or your family, this book and its philosophy are not for you. These are very dangerous tools as they give people an extremely false sense of security with a twisted self-defense mindset that puts them in a poor position of defending themselves. First off, pepper sprays and stun guns while very effective if you are sitting in your living room relaxing, but they are very unreliable at stopping a determined assailant, though not freely available in India, but it can always be imported. Secondly, you have to be in close range to use these tools. With pepper spray you have more distance, but you can't be too far away and hopefully the wind isn't blowing in your direction. With a stun gun you are in hand to hand combat range. The assailant can punch your face in or stab you to death while you are trying to "stun" him. Some shoot a little dart but not only does that have to get through clothing but hopefully you won't miss. Imagine that. And then it's got to work. Thirdly as you are relying on these tools as your means of defense, you have to be able to get to them in time to use them and if they don't work, "highly probable against a determined assailant" then you have no self-defense skills to rely on.

8. KEYS: You also have keys that you carry with you. Keys are basically a small metal stick that you hold in your hand when striking. First, of course you need the item in hand to be of value. Secondly, without hand to hand combat skills you are again relying on something that doesn't mean much in defending you.

9. CONCLUSION ABOUT USE OF WEAPONS: Once you understand how to use your body properly without weapons, you will not only then understand about weapons use, but you will also be able to use weapons much more effectively and to your advantage. In this manual, you will learn how to effectively utilize weapons as an extension of your unarmed combat skills.

10. NO BODYGUARD, NO WEAPONS, and JUST YOUR BODY: Okay now let's get down to totally unarmed hand to hand combat. It's not fun, it's not pleasant, and it's very frightening and very deadly. First off all, are you a tough guy or gal? Seriously, do you have any fighting skills or experience at all? If not, obviously training is important if you care about your self-defense.

❑   ❑   ❑

This page intentionally left blank

Chapter 2

Psychological Aspects of Self Defense

*Knowing when not to fight back
is an important part of Self Defense.*

Psychological Aspects of Self Defense

In any self defense situation, your goal is not to maim or kill your assailant. It is rather to stay alive, and survive a desperate confrontation. If flight is possible, escape by any means. If you are trapped, be prepared to fight. Proper application of deadly force may represent the only viable means by which the intended victim can expect to have a chance of living through an assault by an aggressively determined, physically powerful, possibly armed attacker. Before using Self Defense for personal protection, quickly determine if the following three conditions exist:

1. By means of their language, actions, behavior, or demeanor, another person has demonstrated their intent to kill or severely injure you;

2. This person has the means at hand to carry out their intent, because they are armed with a knife, gun, club, or other lethal weapon, or, if unarmed, they are physically capable of overpowering you;

3. The physical conditions of the encounter are such that the other person has the opportunity to carry out the attack.

These conditions warrant the use of deadly force on your part. Keep in mind that all three criteria must exist. Such conduct is not warranted merely to protect property. You must, unequivocally, be in fear of your life.

Physiology/Psychology of a Fight:

In Self-defense, preparedness and practice are paramount. Be alert. When outside the home, the importance of maintaining an awareness of one's physical surroundings is obvious, with increased vigilance required under unfamiliar or suspect conditions. In a like manner, it is just as important to understand and anticipate the instinctual alarm reactions your mind and body will likely assume in the event you ever experience a violent attack. In a life threatening situation, the intended victim's "fight or flight" reflex manifests itself. This reflex, honed by millenniums of adaptive human survival behavior, results in increased heart rate and cardiac output, higher blood pressure, accelerated respiration, greater carbohydrate metabolism, and virtually instantaneous supercharging of the body.

This stimulation is attributable to the adrenal glands above the kidneys which produce steroidal hormones, and the hormones and neurotransmitters epinephrine (adrenaline) and norepinephrine, responsible for constricting blood vessels and dilating bronchi in the lungs. The stress, rage, and fear which overwhelm the intended victim thus create a bodily alarm reaction which expresses itself as a period of greater strength and faster speed, accompanied by near impervious reaction to pain. At the same time, fine motor skills grossly deteriorate, dexterity noticeably decreases, and the hands, arms and legs may tremble. The intended victim will also likely experience an altered state of perception as well. One, indeed, is not calm, cool and collected. The perception of time may become distorted. With the body alarm reaction, the mind processes stimuli at a fantastically accelerated rate when compared to normal. The result may be the perception that activities are occurring in slow motion, even though movements of the event may actually be extremely fast. The reverse may also occur, the event may seem to transpire faster than one would expect. In its in incredibly heightened state of awareness, the mind of the intended victim tends to focus with tunnel vision on the identified threat. This results in the exclusion of normal peripheral vision. Knowledge of this potential visual reaction to an attack is valuable in the event one is ever faced with multiple assailants. The perception of hearing, like vision, may also be drastically affected during a life threatening encounter. The mind screens out everything that is extraneous to immediate survival, resulting in auditory exclusion. The distorted perception of hearing may mute shouts, sirens and screams. You may not even hear your own shout. The "fight or flight" reflex allows the mind to draw upon memory resources that are not normally used.

The intended victim may experience a sense of precognition, an anticipation response to a subconsciously perceived sequence of circumstances. You "see it coming", even though to the casual observer no violent threat as yet exists. Be prepared to experience a denial response to a life or death situation. One tends to seek mental and emotional shelter in normalcy. When this state of mind is horrifically shattered, the intended victim's reaction may be "this can't be happening". One may experience "hysterical blindness" during or after an attack. Essentially, the mind refuses to visualize any longer a terrifying event perceived by the eyes. This may translate into fleeing the scene of an attack, even if one successfully, and legally, used lethal force to survive the incident. In a highly trained person who has practiced to a degree that the body's reaction to a stimulus is automatic, the "fight or flight" reflex may create the illusion of "watching one's self ". The body movement is so fast, without the guidance of deliberate thought that one's conscious mind can't keep up. The highest manifestation of the phenomenon of observing oneself occurs as an "out of body" experience. Due to trauma, the mind's survival instinct drives all senses into a state of profound and unparalleled perception. From sounds and recalled sights, the mind is able to generate three dimensional images. The "out of body" experience is often combined with a tunnel of white light. It may be experienced by those clinically dead, who miraculously recover, as well as by those victims of an attack who believe them to be mortally wounded, near imminent death. After a life threatening encounter, the intended victim may occasionally revert to a state similar to that of sleep walking, seeming to be in a zombie-like trance.

Confusion is a state of mind commonly experienced by an intended victim who has survived a life or death encounter. Manifestations include remembering events out of sequence, exaggerating the importance of trivial incidents, and forgetting important events due to short term memory loss. The ramifications of the foregoing physical-psychological aspects of encountering, enduring, and evading a life threatening violent attack is obvious: recognize in yourself how your body and mind may react, and prepare yourself accordingly to the extent possible. Mental preparedness is one aspect of self defense. Likewise, it is apparent that an intended victim who has survived a violent encounter is not going to be in the best frame of mind to immediately recount details of the incident to law enforcement authorities. Physically, the adrenalin rush which supercharged the body has given way to a precipitous decline in energy, and the intended victim is likely exhausted and confused. For these reasons, it is not a good idea to give legal statements regarding an attack right away, especially if the attack was terminated by the justifiable use of deadly force on your part. Rather, politely advise the police officers that you understand your rights. Then get some rest, collect your thoughts, and consult with an attorney.

Tips for effective Self Defense Techniques:

1. **Be willing to act:** Your chance for success is determined by your attitude. If attacked, fight back. If someone has to be hurt, let it be the attacker.

2. **Don't be an easy victim:** Shout! Resist! Fight!

3. **Element of Surprise:** As soon as you shout and resist, the element of surprise is on your side. Your attacker does not expect effective resistance. Distract him – Move quickly and keep using defensive tactics until you control the situation.

4. **Develop Self Confidence:** Believe in your own ability to use the Self Defense techniques. Practice until your response is instinctive.

5. **Believe in what you are doing:** Act with determination – Simple Self Defense techniques does work, and they will work for you.

6. **Don't Panic:** If you can't control yourself, you can't control the situation.

7. **Bluff:** Make an effort to show your attacker you are not afraid – concentrating on wining.

8. **Escape:** Your first inclination may be to run. But run only if there is a safe place nearby where other people can help you. If there is nobody to help you, run only after you have made sure the attacker cannot pursue.

9. **Keep it Simple:** You are not out to dazzle anyone with a slick routine. Stick to only those technique which you can use easily and quickly.

10. **Don't Hesitate:** Once you are forced to defend yourself, use everything available to you; Shout, Strike, Kick, Bite, and Throw something. If you start a defense, finish it.

11. **Don't Depend on Bye-standers for Help:** People watching you being attacked may help you or may not help you. Be confident, trust yourself and fight with spirit and determination.

12. **Know Yourself:** Don't have two strangers to deal with in the attack. Know yourself and your capabilities. Be prepared to use everything you know you can do, and if that is not enough, be prepared to improvise.

13. **Never Fight an Opponent unless forced to:** If your attacker is only after your money or any other personal property, give it to him. Do not risk your life to save money.

14. **Don't expect to fight gently:** An attacker is no gentleman.

Precautionary measures for effective Self Defense:

Awareness of facts is the key to prevention. Women, children, and men, of all ages, socioeconomic levels, neighborhoods and lifestyles can be assaulted. Assailants look for available vulnerable targets. 85% of all rape victims know or at least are familiar with their assailants.

- Be especially aware of your surroundings at times when you may be less alert and more vulnerable to an attack, e.g., during exams, when you are upset, sick, tired, or when you have been drinking.

- Use discretion and caution when taking shortcuts through isolated parts.

- If you must be in an isolated area, e.g., working or studying alone in labs or offices, lock the doors and tell a friend or security where you are and when you plan to return.

- Know the location of emergency phones on routes to and from class.

- Keep personal belongings in view.

- Wherever you are, if you see or hear someone who might be in trouble, your options include running, yelling, confronting, and calling the police.

While Using ATM Machines:

- If you feel threatened while using the ATM, push the cancel button to cancel your transaction. Just walk away and complete your transaction later.

- Avoid using an ATM at night. Most ATM crimes occur between 7:00 p.m. and midnight.

- If you must use an ATM at night, take another person with you.

- Check around the ATM first to make sure no one is lurking in the shadows.

- Use machines that can be clearly seen from the street or public area.

- Use machines that are in well-lighted areas.

While at Home:

- Install and use locks on your doors and windows

- Have your locks changed, re-keyed or add a new lock when you move into a new house or apartment.

- Keep doors locked day or night whether you are at home or not.

- Know who is at the door before opening it. Demand I.D.'s from anyone you don't know.

- If someone comes to your door and asks to use your phone to call for help, offer instead to make the call.

- Close your blinds and shades at night.

- Give your home a "someone home" look. Put radio and lights on a timer.

- Have good lighting around entrances.

- Develop an escape plan for use in case of an intruder or fire.

- Leave spare keys with a friend, not in accessible places.

- Know your neighbors and know which ones you can trust in an emergency.

- Keep emergency numbers near the phone.

- Keep mobile phone charged at all times.

On the Street while Walking:

- Act confident. Look and be alert about the people around you.
- Be aware of your surroundings. Cross the street or change direction if you think you are being followed.
- Be careful when people ask you for directions. Reply from a distance rather than getting too close to the car.
- Travel with a friend whenever possible to reduce the chances of being attacked. This includes going to public restrooms.
- Wear clothes and shoes that give you freedom of movement.
- Vary your route if possible.
- Notice cars that pull up beside you or pass you more than once.
- Keep one hand free when walking.
- Carry change for bus fare or a telephone call.
- Do not hesitate to get attention however you can if you are in trouble. Do not be afraid to make a scene.
- If you travel a regular route at night, become familiar with stores that stay open, gas stations, and other places where there will be people.

While Driving a Car:

- Have your keys in your hand as you approach the car.
- Lock your doors when driving and after parking.
- Check the back seat and floor.
- Always keep at least half a tank of fuel in your car.
- Maintain the car in good running condition.
- Keep your valuables out of sight, under the seat, in the glove compartment or trunk.
- Avoid parking next to vans, as you can be pulled in through the sliding door.
- Should another motorist offer to help, roll down window only an inch and ask him or her to call the police?
- Keep emergency kits containing a flashlight, telephone change, distress signs, and other essentials in your car.

On the Telephone:

- Be wary of telephone surveys.
- List only your first initial and last name in the telephone directory.
- Think about the information you give out over the telephone and to people you don't know well. Tell roommates and housemates not to give information by phone about who is home, who is out, how long anyone is expected to be out.
- Never reveal your number to a wrong number caller.
- If you receive a threatening or obscene phone call, hang up, contact the police and

make a report.

- Answering machines may be used to screen calls. Your outgoing message should not say that you are away from home.

On an Elevator:

- Check the inside of an elevator before entering. Wait for the next elevator if you are unsure of the people inside.
- When riding an elevator, stand by the control board. If you feel in danger, press all the buttons and get off the elevator as soon as possible.

On Public Transportation:

- Check the bus schedule to avoid long waits at the bus stop. Become familiar with routes and time tables in your area.
- Wait for buses at well-lighted stops.
- If possible, join other people at a nearby stop.
- If someone bothers you on the bus, say loudly, "Leave me alone!" or "No!" Get up and find another seat. Tell the driver.
- Stay awake on public transportation if you are alone.
- Notice, who else gets off at your stop. If you feel someone is following you, walk towards a populated area. Avoid walking directly home.
- Be aware that hitchhiking can be very dangerous.

While Cycling:

- Use reflectors, reflective tape, or other similar devices on cycling shoes, fenders, belts, frames, pedals and handlebars.
- Keep to the left. Ride with traffic, not against it.
- Use hand signals to indicate turning or stopping.
- Walk your bicycle across busy intersections.
- Avoid cycling in bad weather.
- Perform regular maintenance checks.
- Secure it properly with chains and locks.
- Report any suspicious person you may see loitering around bicycle racks.

While Jogging:

- Be aware of your environment.
- If you feel insecure about defending yourself, consider jogging with a friend.
- Choose well-traveled running paths and be aware of any isolated areas you will run through. Vary your route.
- At night, wear light-colored clothing or reflective markings.
- Tell your family members or another friend your route and expected time of return.

- If approached by a car while running alone, do not stop to give directions or answer questions. Leave the road and head for a populated area.
- Don't let yourself be surprised. Listening to your headset may make you unable to hear approaching traffic, emergency sirens or any other danger signals.

If Attacked...Self Defense:

- If someone tries to snatch your purse, let it go. Most injuries from robberies occur during purse snatches when people resist.
- If you are attacked, whether you resist and how you resist will depend on your personal resources and your personal values. Give some thought right now to what you would do in various situations that could arise. The more you have thought ahead, the more likely you'll be to act in the way you've planned.
- Have you taken training in self-defense? Do you think you could hit or kick someone who is attacking you?
- Do you know how to get away from someone grabbing you? What objects could you use to defend yourself?
- In considering your reactions to different situations, keep these three basic rules in mind:
  1. Trust your instincts.
  2. Don't be afraid to be impolite or make a scene; this is especially important, even if it is someone you know.
  3. Try to remain calm-use your imagination and good judgment; give yourself time to think.

Victim's Rights:

- You have the right to ask questions of the police, doctors, attorneys, counselors or agencies, so that you understand.
- You have the right to be treated in a considerate and sensitive manner by law enforcement personnel.
- It is normal to feel fear, anger, loneliness and helplessness.
- It is normal to act non-emotional, non-feeling or hysterical, but don't put others to inconvenience.
- It is normal-and often healthy-to cry.

You have the right to report the attack to law enforcement and expect that all avenues within the law will be pursued to apprehend and convict the offender.

❑ ❑ ❑

Chapter 3
Exercises for Fitness

An ounce of practice is worth several tons of theory.

Exercises for Fitness

The human body requires constant exercise; and regular exercise aids digestion, stimulates circulation and helps the body to resist diseases. We are what we ingest! Our environment is polluted. Our air and food are full of chemical wastes, preservatives and additives which affect our personalities. Hypertension and heart disease cause more deaths per year than any other accidents. As modern people, we must learn to survive these obstacles; we all have basically the same equipment; heart, lungs, kidneys, liver, spleen, pancreas and other organs necessary for life support. Our bodies are delicate machines that need daily maintenance. Food is our fuel, legs are our suspension system, hearts and lungs are our compressors, brain, which is the bio-computer, controls all of the body's logic and behavioral programming. Our brain is capable of storing vast amount of data. How we think and what we eat affect our personality. Our life support systems are a combination of three basic mechanisms, the bio-computer, compressor, and the suspension system. Exercise and nutrition are necessary to maintain the proper balance between the bio-computer and the other two systems.

Our body resembles a rubber band. If left inactive, it will contract and soon become stiff and brittle, any sudden or violent motion can cause it to snap, resulting in serious injury. Moderation is the key word, to proceed gradually step-by-step. The intensity of the exercise should only be increased once the body is flexible enough to withstand the heightened tension without risking unnecessary strains or pulls. Remember we are not too old, to exempt ourselves from any exercise program no matter what age it may be. The body that remains supple is able to endure the pressure of everyday living. Keep the body in shape, not merely toned but beyond the point of barely making it, you will notice a marked improvement in the body and also harmony with your surrounding environment.

I Limbering Exercises:

Neck:

a)

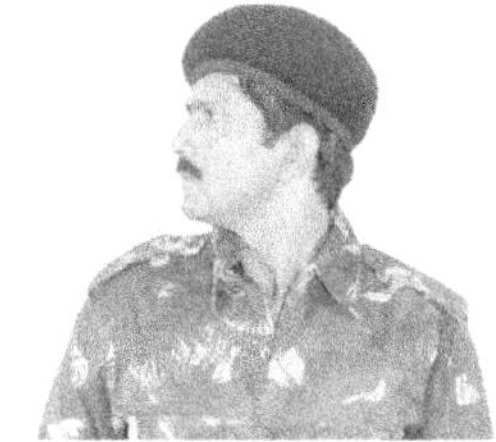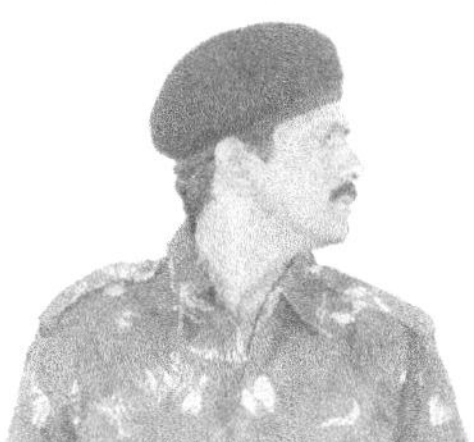

Twist head side to side – 20 counts.

b)

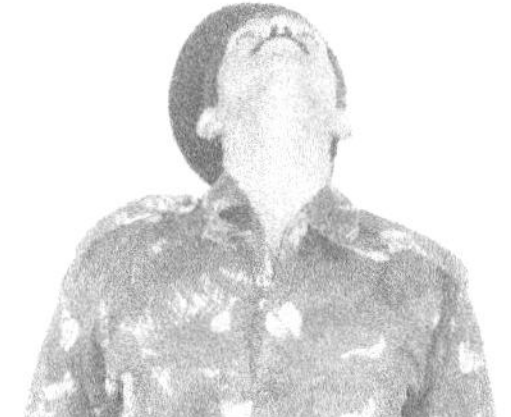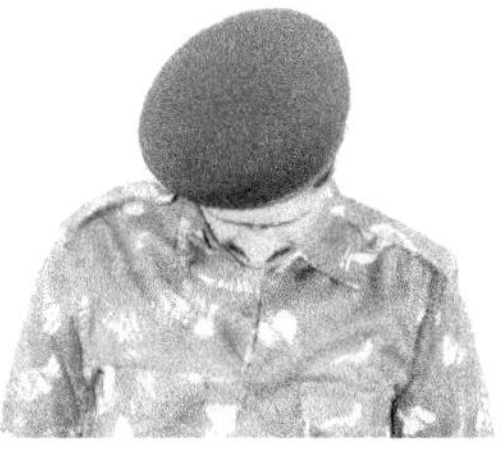

Raise the head high up and lower it down
till the chin touches the hollow of throat -20 counts.

c)

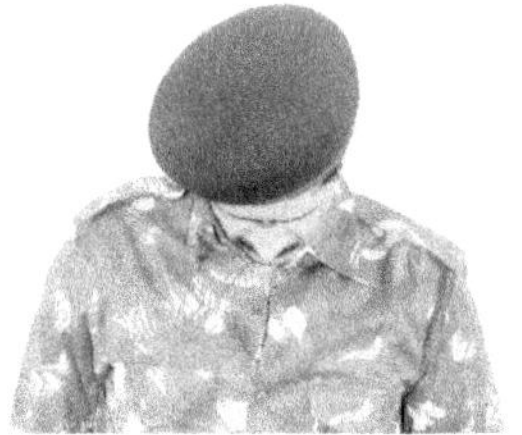

Rotate head in all four direction, first clockwise for 10 counts
& then anticlockwise for another 10 counts.

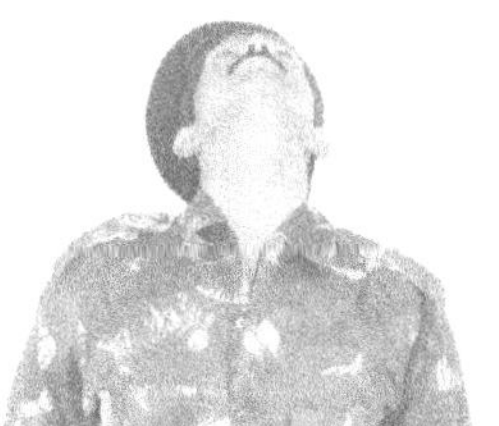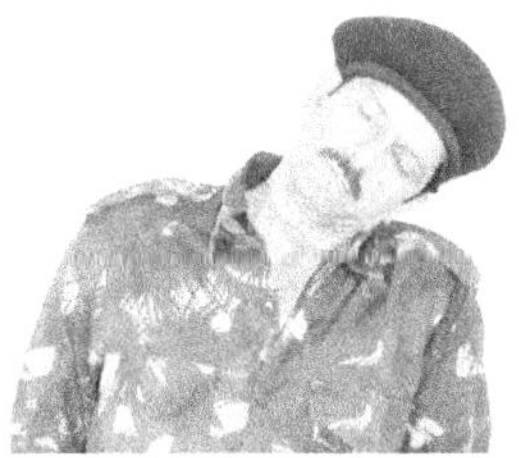

Shoulders & Arms:

a) Arm Swinging

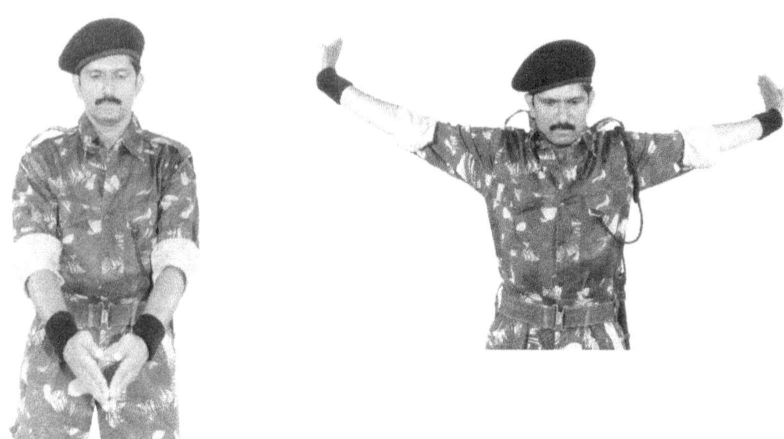

Raise arms from waist level and then stretch to ear level, keeping elbow joints straight and wrist joints bend at right angle from behind – 20 counts.

b) Circling the Shoulder

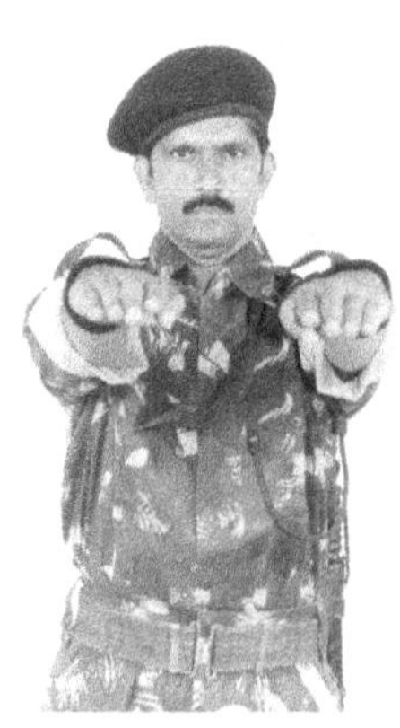

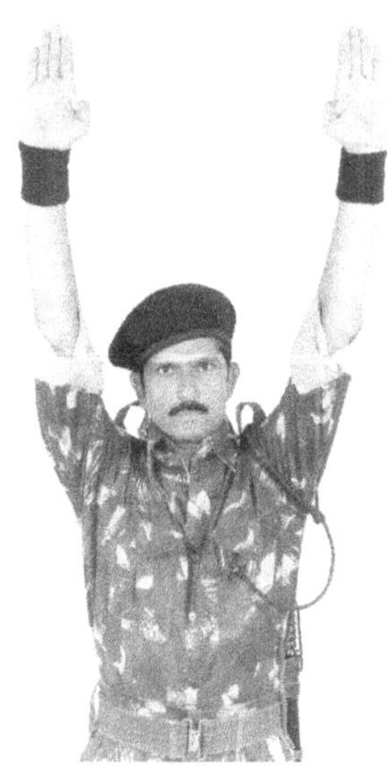

From shoulder level rotate the hand fully in a circle in clockwise direction for 10 counts and then rotate anticlockwise – 10 counts.

Waist & Hips:

a) Twisting

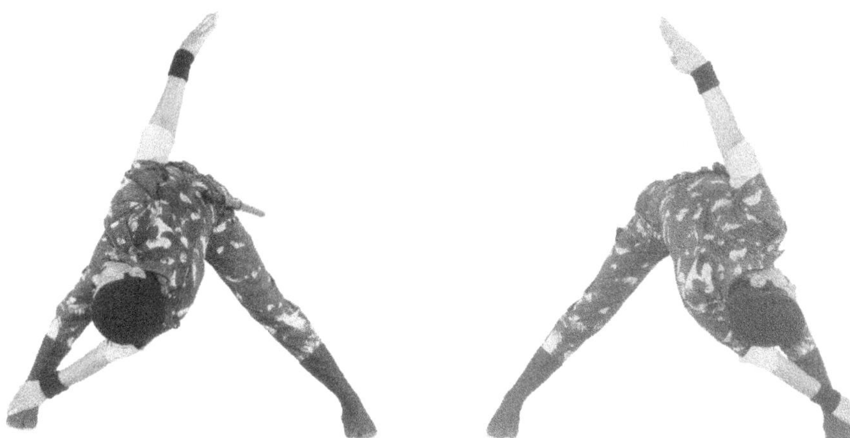

Spread the legs, double shoulder length, bend the body forward, keep the knees locked, then touch the right toe with the left hand and left toe with the right hand – 20 counts.

b) Front Bending

Stand with feet together, knees locked. Bend the waist, and then try to touch your forehead to the knees, without bending the knees, gradually try to touch your chin to the knees - 20 counts.

Repeat the same exercise in sitting position, hands holding the ankle, chest touching the thighs and chin trying to touch the knee, without bending the knee - 20 counts

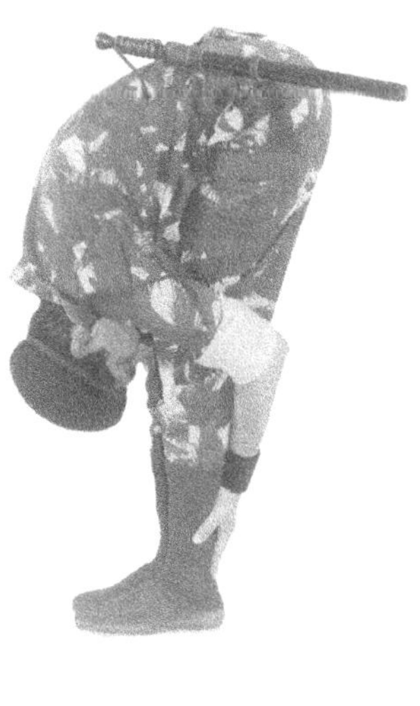

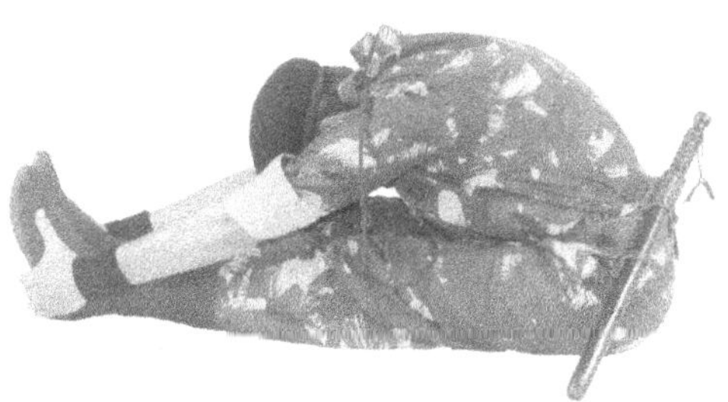

c) Side Bending

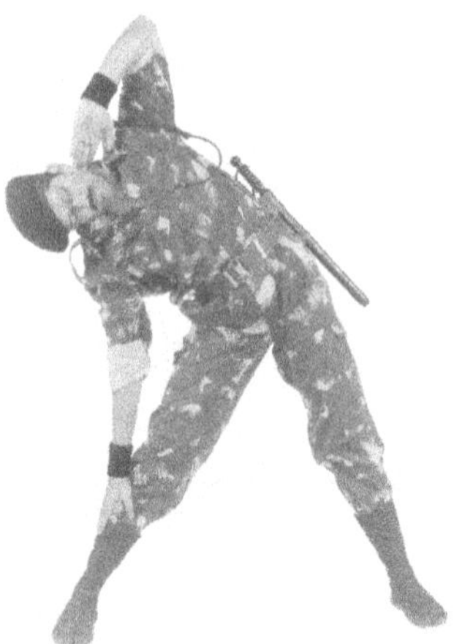 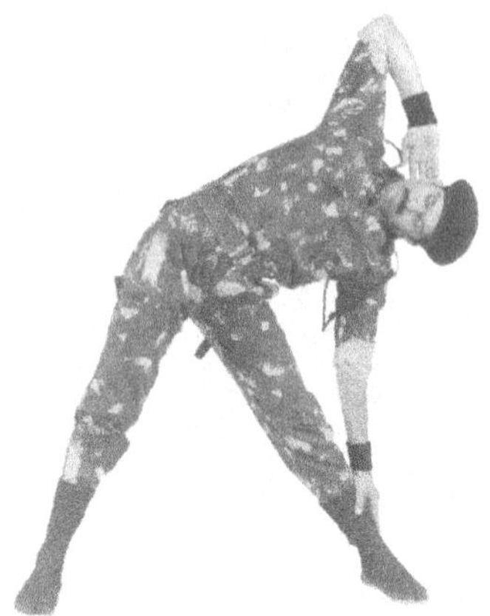

Stand with feet apart, knees locked , bend the waist from side and try to touch your right fingertips to the right side of the right leg, below the knee level, repeat this same procedure for the left side, do this exercise - 20 counts

d) Back Bending

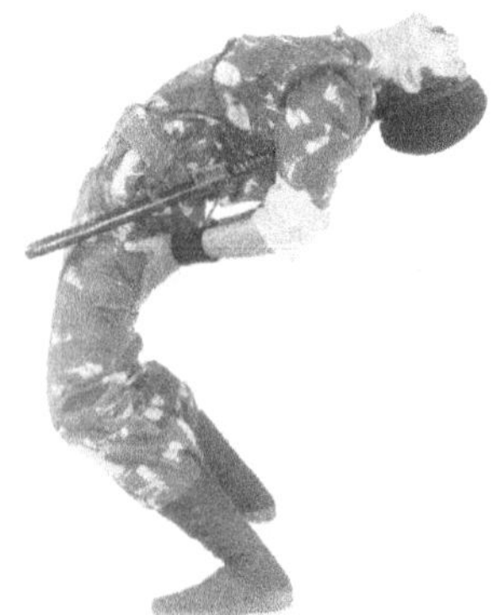 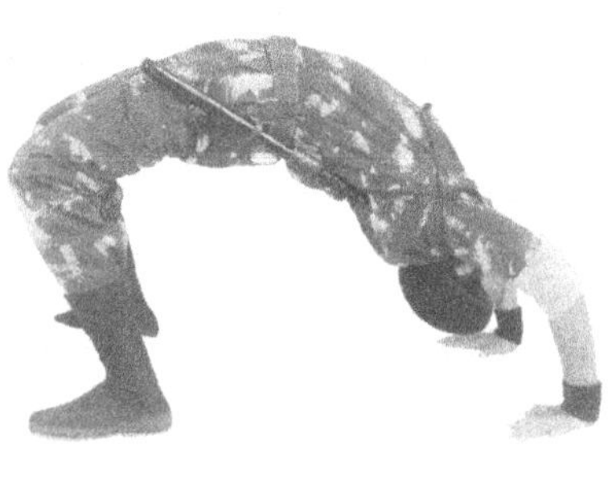

Stand straight, feet spread shoulder distance, bend the waist backward, so much so, that the hands touches the floor from behind, with knees slightly bend - 10 counts.

Legs:

a) Leg Swinging

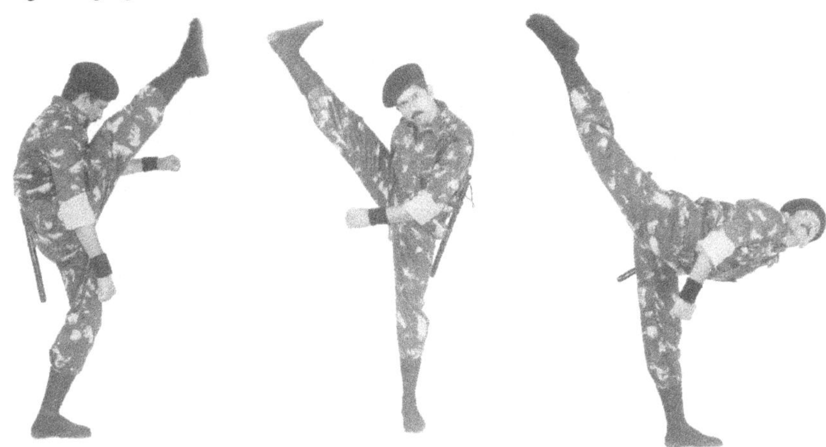

Swing the legs in front, side, back position, without bending the knees of the swinging leg and try to maintain the balance, the balancing leg's heel should not be lifted above the ground. Do this exercise for 20 counts

b) Ankle Twisting

In standing position, keep your hands on the head, then try to raise both the toes without bending the knee, while standing on the heels. Then get the toes down, raise the heels and squat a little with knees bent, do it alternatively - 20 counts.

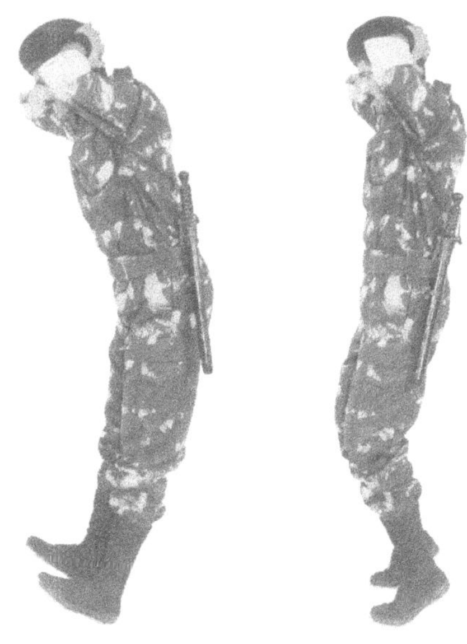

II Strengthening Exercises:

a) Push-ups

Sit down with feet together and knees together, with knees touching the floor, then place palms on outside of knees, this becomes the distance between the two hands. Now stretch the legs behind and keep it together, knees locked. At this juncture, the full body weight is on the two palms and balls of the feet of two legs, which is in contact with the floor. Waist firm and tight, in line with feet & shoulder, as shown in the figure. Now go down, touch your forehead and chest and come up the same way. Remember, only the forehead and chest touches the floor and nothing else (except palms and feet also touch the ground). While coming up, let the whole body come up, including the waist, don't allow it to dangle. Let the full body, come up in one piece – 10 minimum.

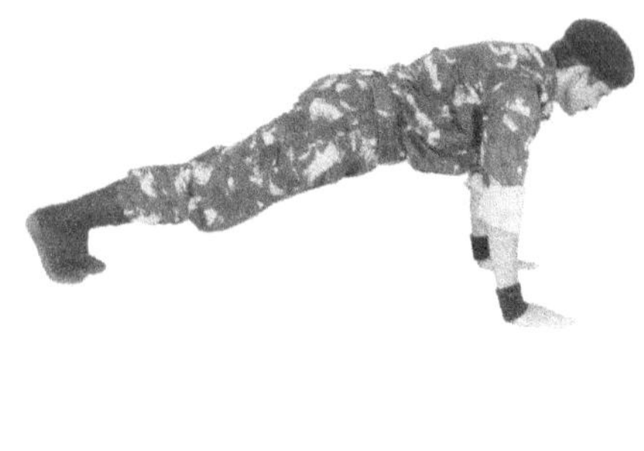

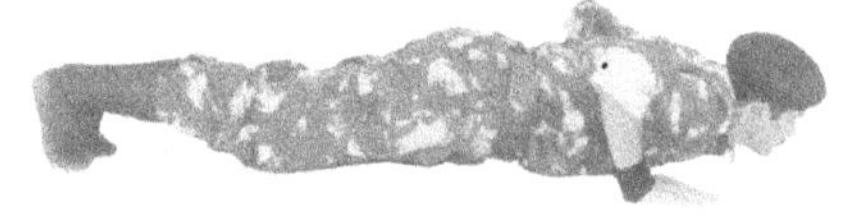

b) Sit-ups

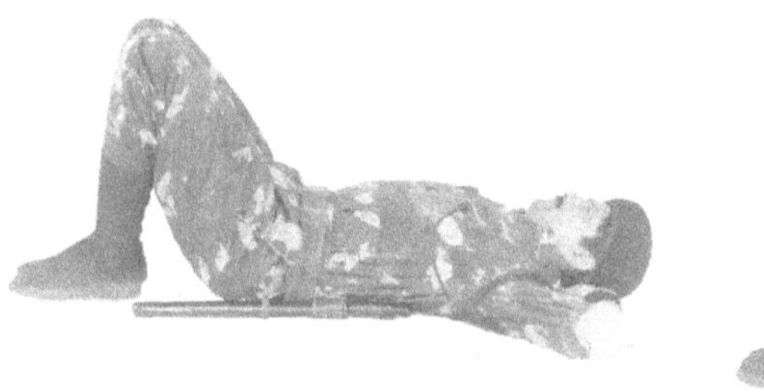

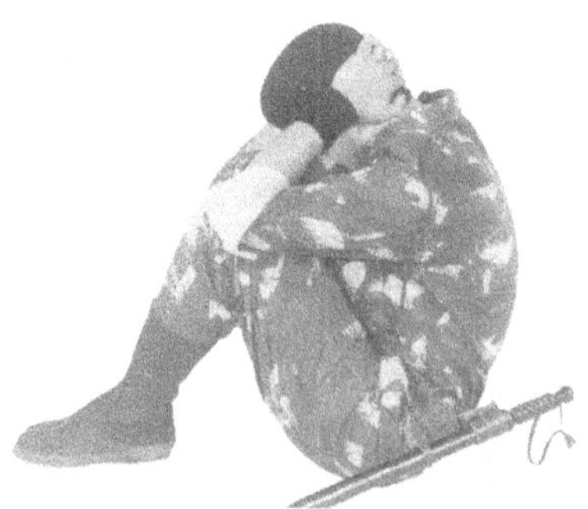

Lie flat on the ground with knees bent and feet together. Hands back of head, lift your head and touch your forehead to your knees, then go back to the starting position, as described above. Do this for 30 counts. Don't move the feet while doing the sit-ups.

c) Squatting

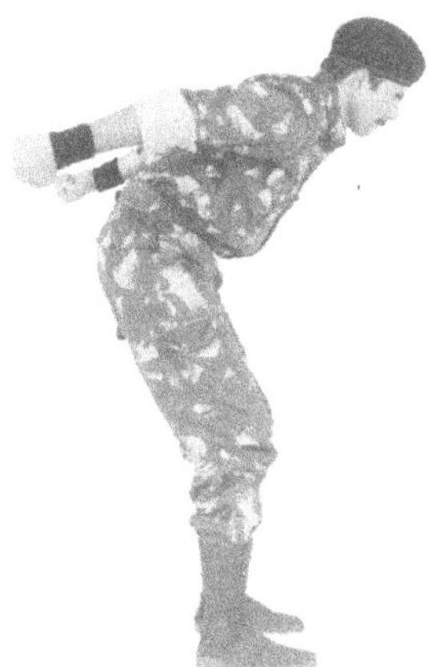

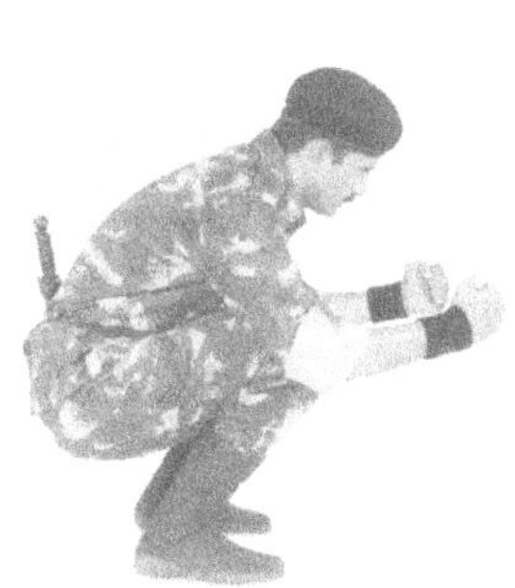

This is the normal Indian baithaks, the hands can be either at the side or on the head, do it for 50 counts.

d) Jogging & Skipping

Jogging could be done in the open space for five to ten minutes.

OR

Skipping with the help of skipping rope for 3 minutes with 3 repetitions can also built your cardiovascular system and gives you enough stamina for your regular day to day activity.

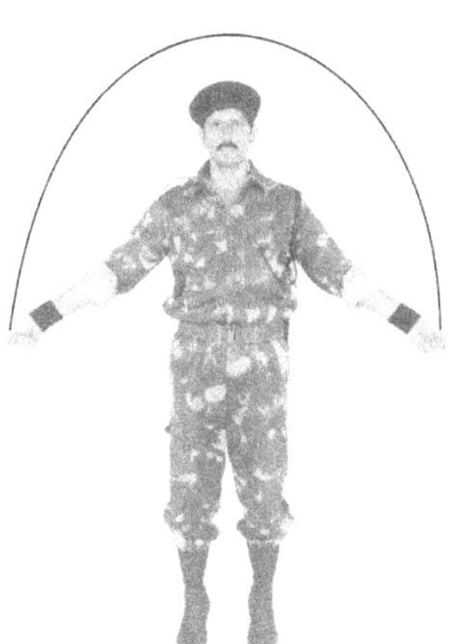

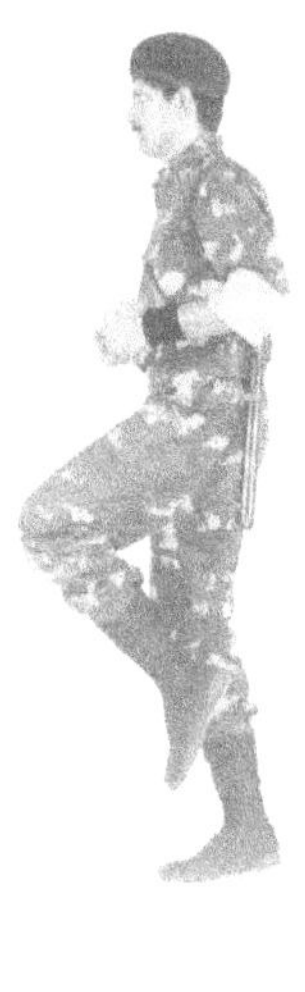

e) Weight Training

i) Alternate Curling

ii) Tricep Extension

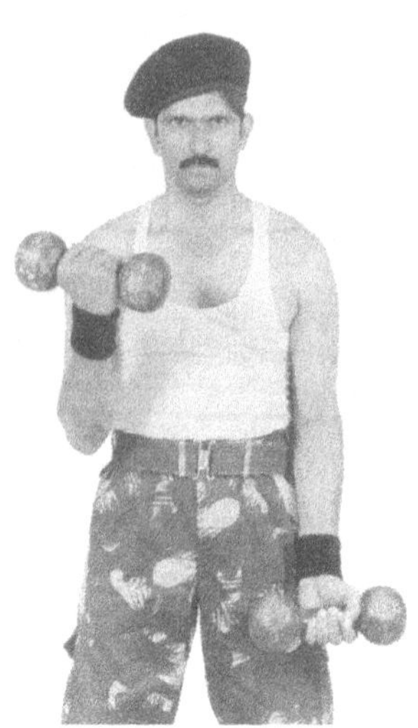

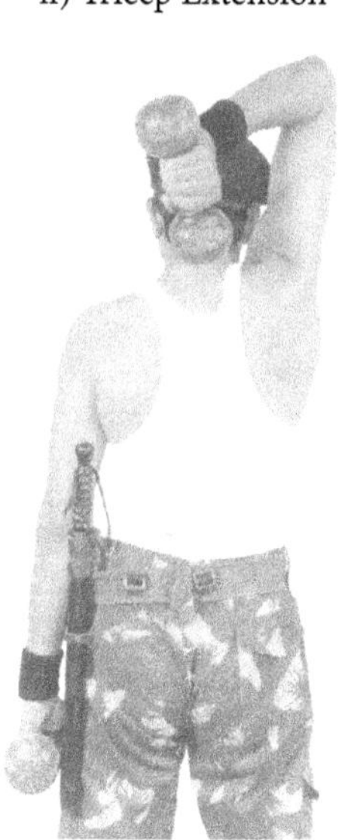

iii) Lateral Shoulder raises

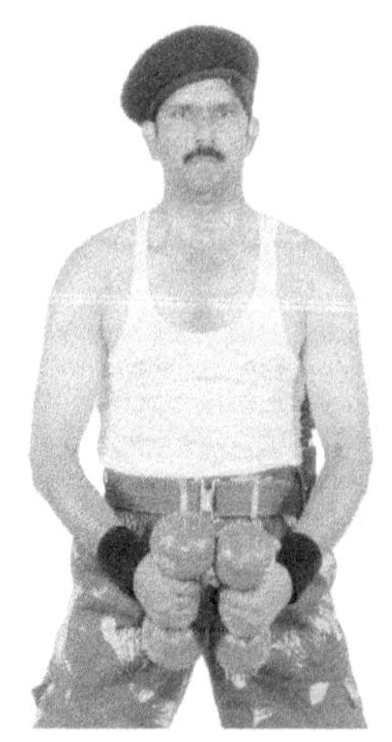

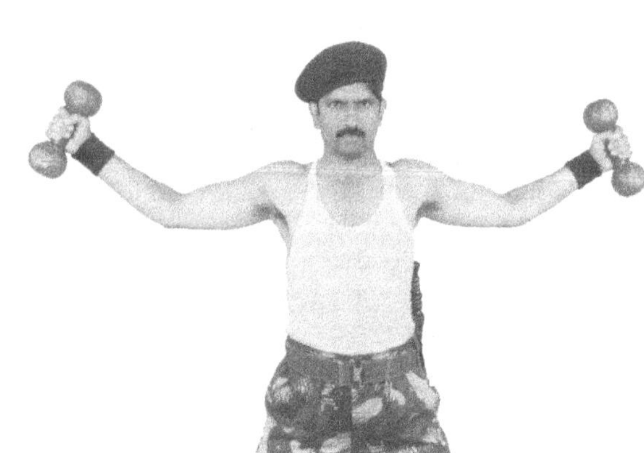

iv) Bent Shoulder raises

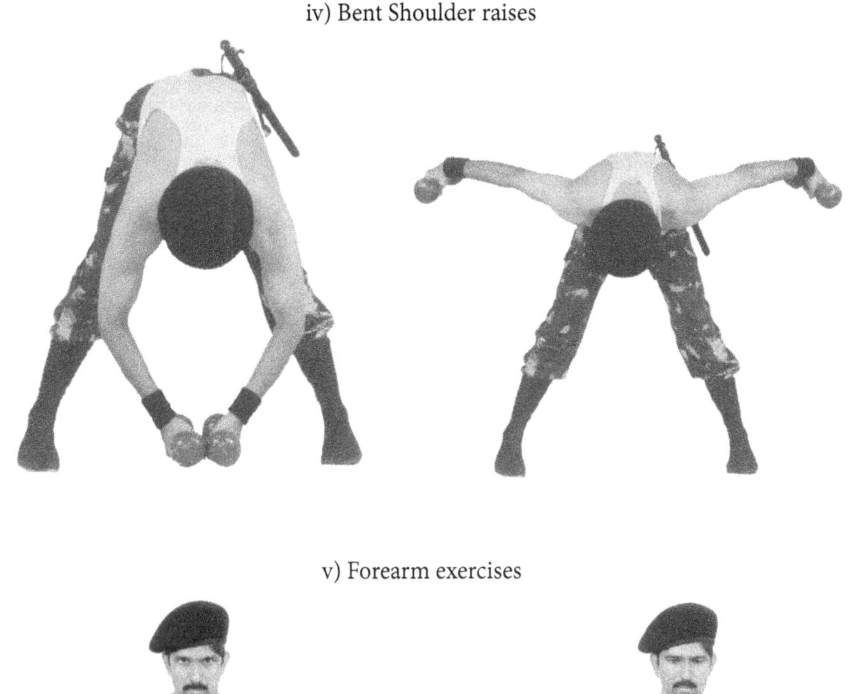

v) Forearm exercises

Weight training exercises can be done according to an each individual needs, a well balanced program could be of 20 repetitions on both sides for minimum three sets. After a month or two one can vary according to each individual's needs.

f) Training with equipment

To sharpen your skill in self defense, you have to train with various equipments. With the world proceeding in the 21st century, so also the equipment in the field of self defense has become highly advanced, scientific, durable, and highly expensive. But many prefer to use the age old method of training equipments, such as the punching bag, punching gloves, kicking pad, etc.

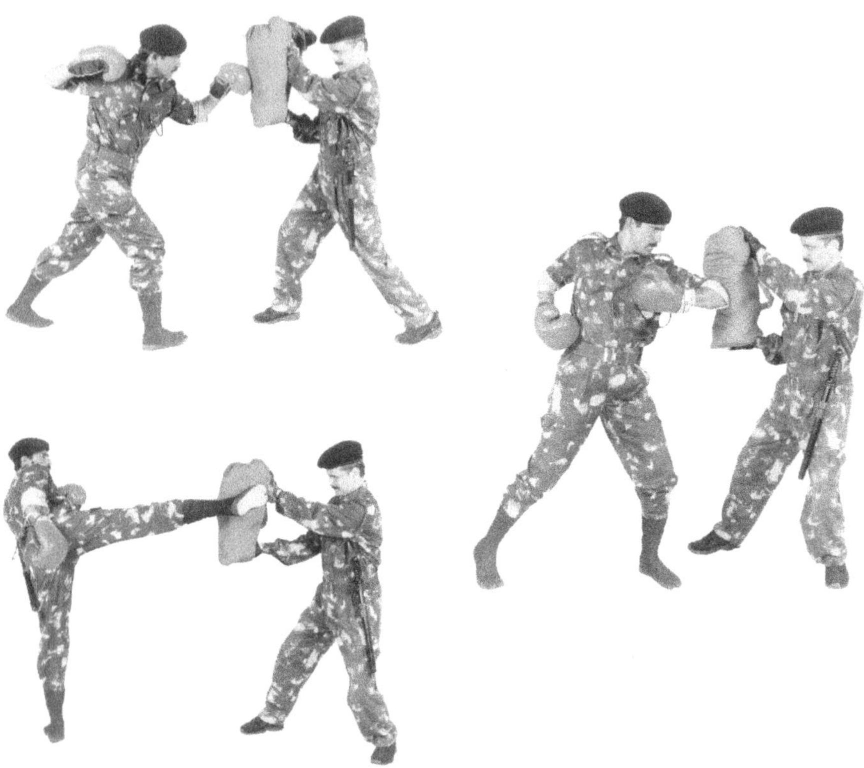

To develop speed and power one can strike a hanging punching bag, or let your partner hold the punching bag for you as shown in the accompanying figure. One can practice full power punching, kicking, or elbow striking techniques. This type of training will help you to understand, how it is the feeling when you strike a real opponent, the only drawback is that real opponent moves in various direction and it can hit back, while punching bag and kicking pad, don't hit back.

g) Shadow Boxing

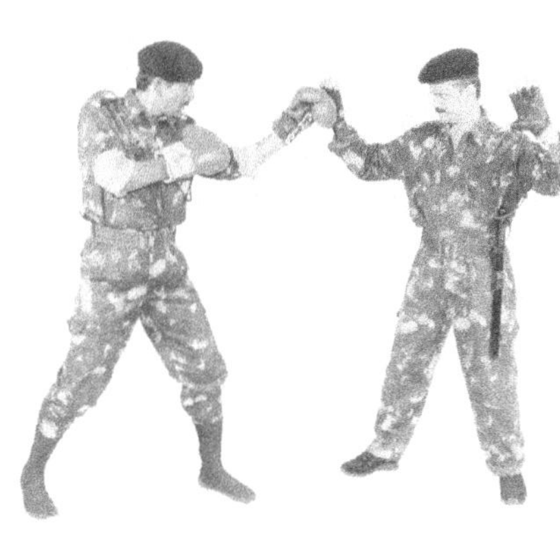

Shadow Boxing plays a crucial part in Self Defense training. Shadow Boxing helps to improve agility, speed, timing, accuracy and focus. It also helps to improve your footwork in a very rhythmic manner, without loosing balance or feeling clumsy about your movement. To avoid injury one can take support from boxing gloves, punching pad or kicking pad, if nothing is available, then the partners palm is more than enough for target practice, but see that you are properly well equipped so as to avoid any injury to the opponent's palm. One can practice a series of punching, kicking or elbow striking techniques, without suffering or loosing balance in a very rhythmic manner.

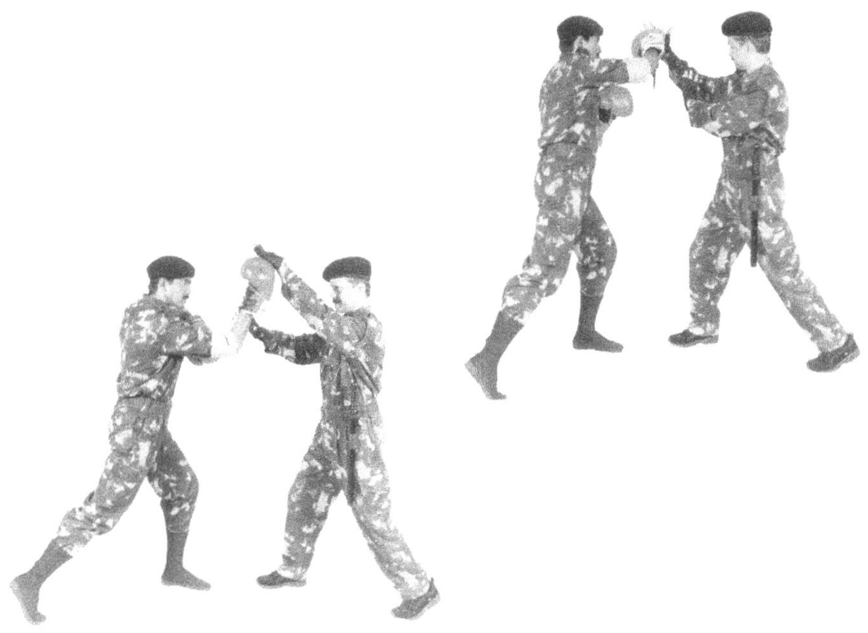

Long Wave Breathing

Stand in a relaxed position, legs-shoulder width distance, knees slightly bent hands at the side and eyes front, mind empty. Concentrate below the navel. Slowly lift your hands up to shoulder height, as though you are lifting a heavy object, palms facing the ceiling, body relaxed. Breathe in the lower lungs, middle and the upper lungs, i.e. abdominal, ribs and chest range respectively by the help of the nose without straining the nostril. The time required to fill the lungs should be equivalent to the time taken to lift the hands up to the shoulder level. Then let the hands come near the chest, wrist touching the chest, palms facing the ceiling, hold the breath for five counts and then, slowly start turning the palms inside and start pressing it downwards towards the hips and simultaneously exhale through the mouth, tongue touching the upper palate and air gushing out forcefully, simultaneously the lungs contract. Body relaxed. Then hold and wait for five counts and restart the cycle for 10 cycles.

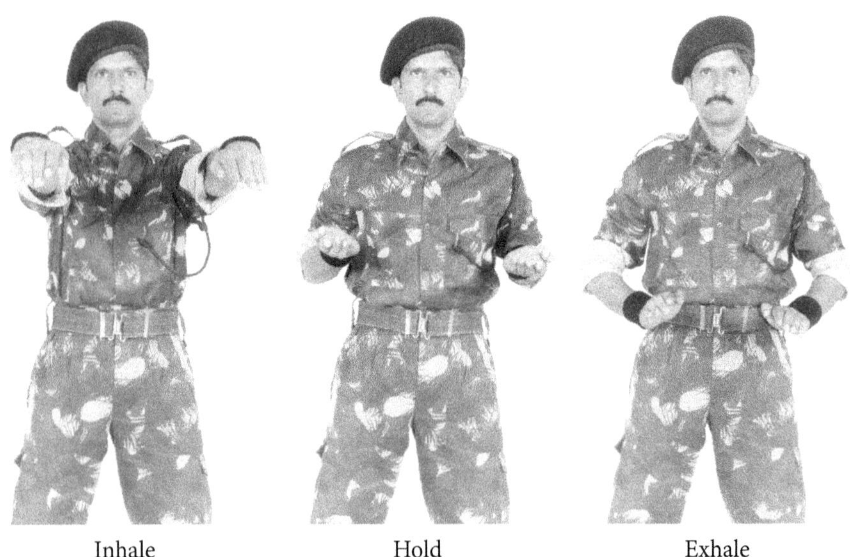

| Inhale | Hold | Exhale |

Benefits: Long wave breathing will help to calm your mind, body and spirit. In times of stress, this breathing is a great rejuvenator.

Chapter 4

Basic Defensive Move

The practice of Self Defense must be Intensive not Extensive

Basic Defensive Move

Dodges play an important role in a combat, with minimum use of energy we can deflect the oncoming blows without any injury to ourselves. Moving out of line of the attack is a simple but very important move which must be practiced countless times so that it becomes virtually automatic. Remember for a successful dodge, one should concentrate well and observe the opponent very closely, as soon as any oncoming blows come, move to dodge, with the help of the moves shown below.

a) Back Dodge

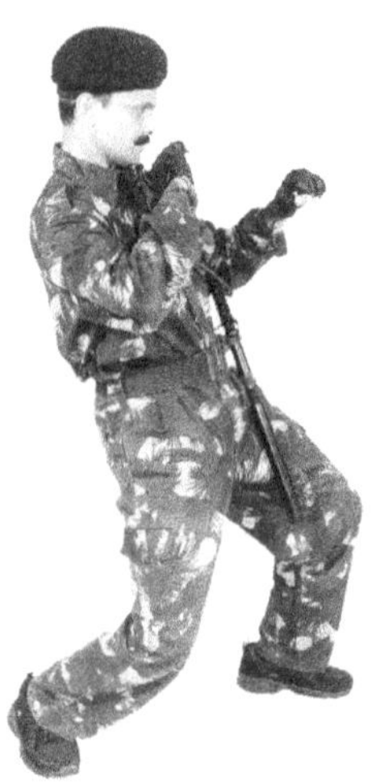 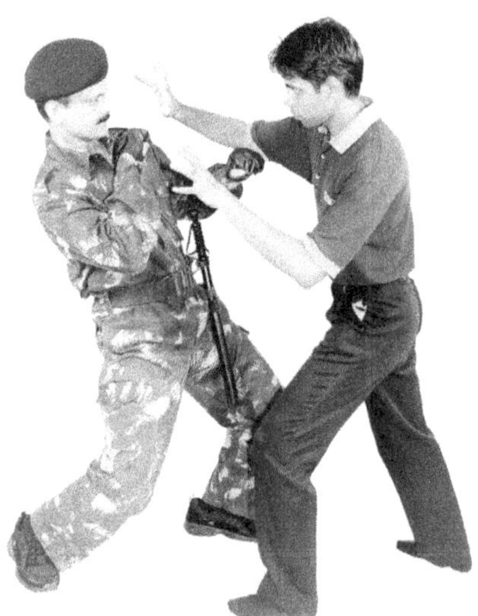

Stand in fighting stance, hands on guard position, eyes on the opponent. Bend your knees, and keep the hip relaxed. As soon as the opponent strikes, start bending backwards, from the waist, till his blow is out of the range. Check one should not loose his balance, and keep a tight vigil on the opponent.

b) Side Dodge

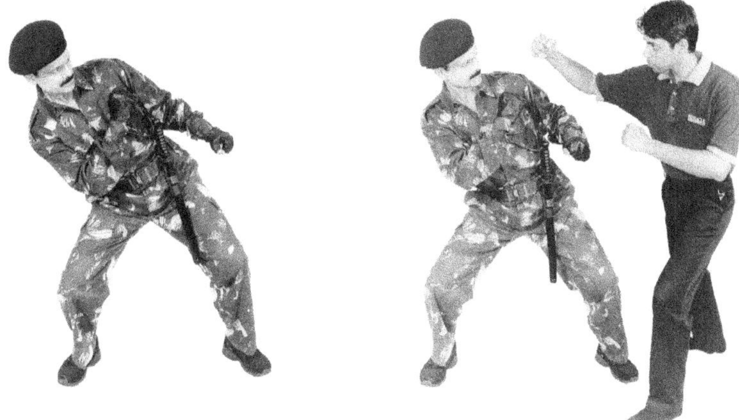

Stand in fighting stance, hands on guard position, eyes on the opponent. Bend your knees, and keep the hip relaxed. As soon as the opponent strikes a roundhouse punch, bend from the waist in sideward direction, till his blow is out of the range. Check one should not loose his balance, and keep an eye on the opponent.

c) Drop Dodge

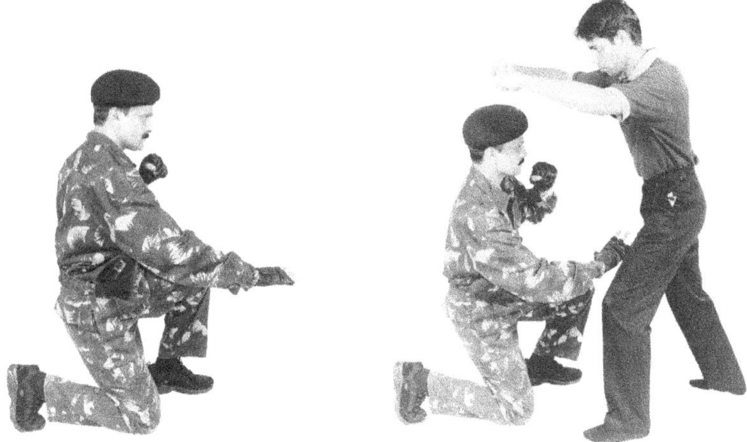

Stand in fighting stance, hands on guard position, eyes on the opponent. Bend your knees, and keep the hip relaxed. As soon as the opponent strikes pull the back leg near the front leg and drop your body down. Your whole body moves in a crouching position, as though it is turned into a ball. Automatically you're out of his striking range and very close to his vulnerable point, i.e. the groin. From this position also keep an eye on the opponent.

II Blocks:

Blocks are used to deflect or guide an oncoming force away from its original path. Your opponent's power is neutralized and diverted to your advantage. The blocking exercises are designed to defend you. As in fencing, you only need to move and block sufficiently out of the line of the attack. If you jump too wide you may be too far away to make your counter-move. Just note the hand or foot of the blocking hand should just skim past you body.

a) Outside Block

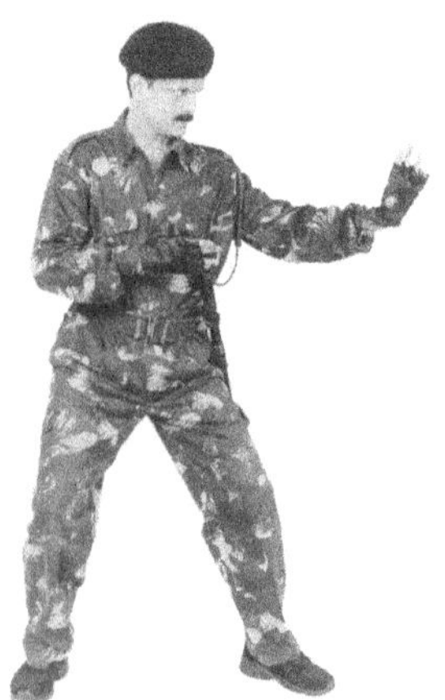 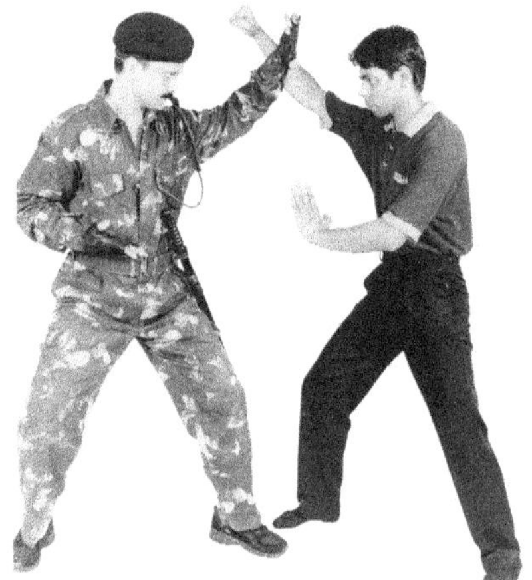

Stand in fighting stance, hands on guard position, eyes on the opponent. Bend your knees, and keep the hip relaxed. As soon as the opponent strikes, let the leading hand move from the rear shoulder and across the solar plexus, chest, and away from the body, till it reaches the extension of the shoulder. (Remember elbow bend). Arm muscles relaxed, but on point of contact against the opponent's limb, tense it, blocking with forearm.

b) Inside Block

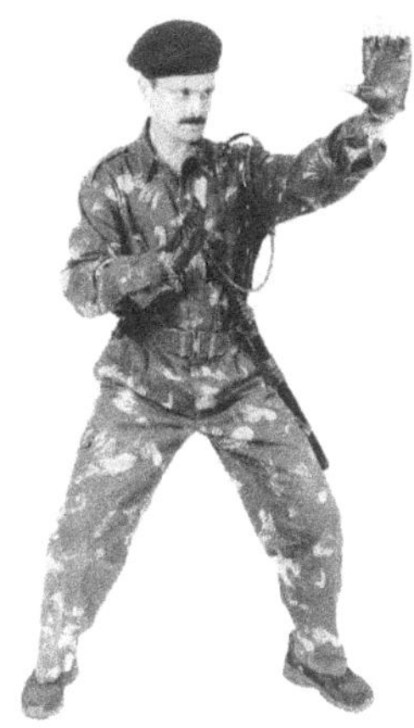 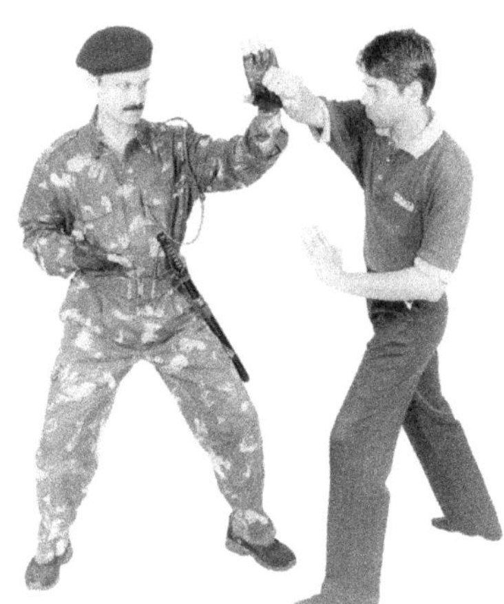

Stand in fighting stance, hands on guard position, eyes on the opponent. Bend your knees, and keep the hip relaxed. As soon as the opponent strikes, let the leading hand move from the leading shoulder towards the solar plexus, and towards the rear shoulder. (Remember elbow bend). Arm muscles relaxed, but on point of contact against the opponent's limb, tense it, blocking with forearm.

c) Rising Block

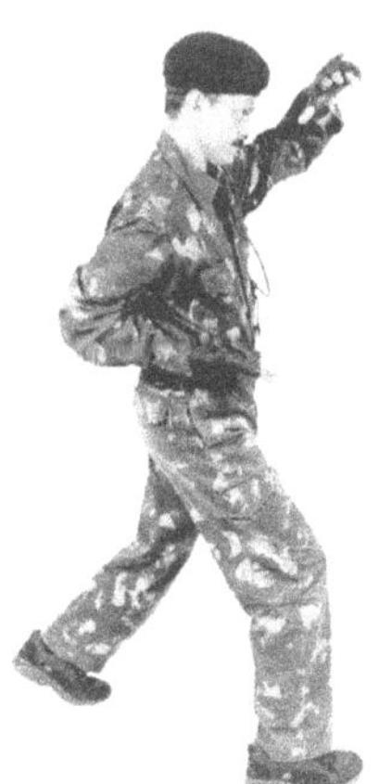 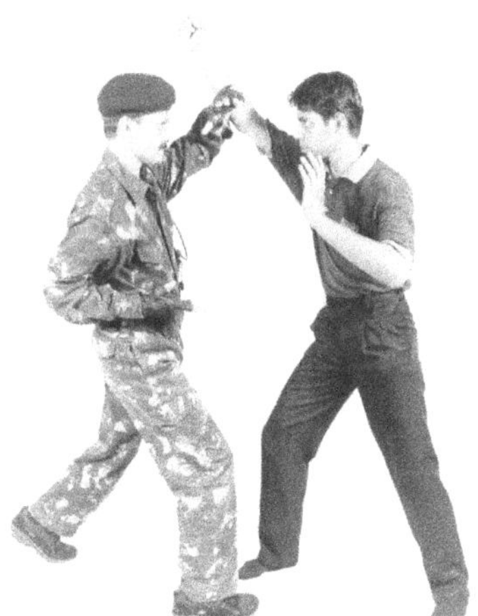

Stand in fighting stance, hands on guard position, eyes on the opponent. Bend your knees, and keep the hip relaxed. As soon as the opponent strikes, let the leading hand move from the waist towards the forehead, traveling across the stomach, chest and forehead, elbows bend at right angle. Forearm parallel to the ground. The block should be done as though lifting the opponent's punch above your forehead. Arm muscles relaxed, but on point of contact against the opponent's limb, tense it, blocking with forearm.

d) Lowering Block

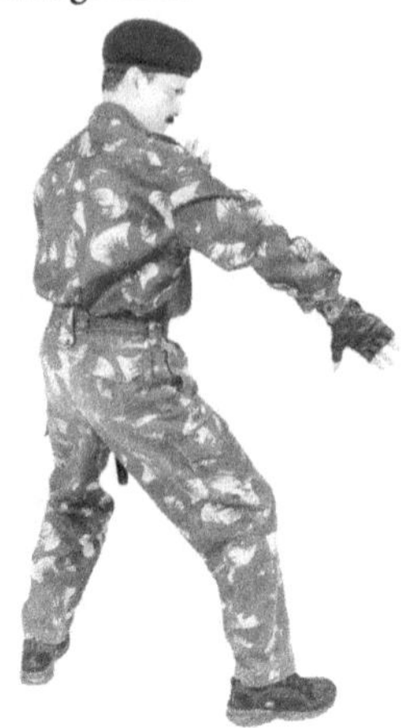 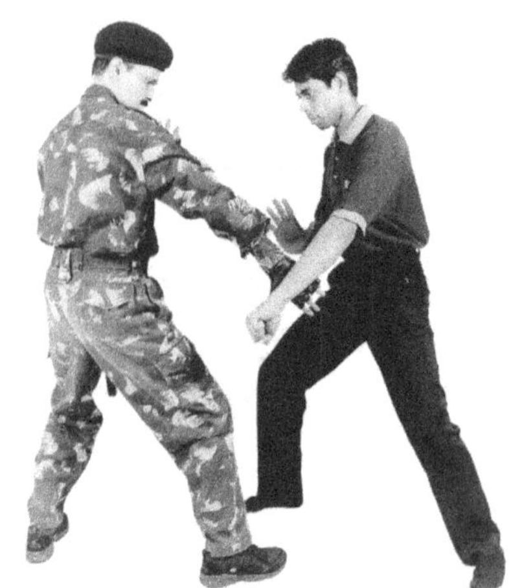

Stand in fighting stance, hands on guard position, eyes on the opponent. Bend your knees, and keep the hip relaxed. As soon as the opponent strikes let the leading hand move from the waist towards the groin across the stomach, elbows bend at right angle. Forearm parallel to the ground. The block should be done as though pressing the opponent's punch towards the ground region. Arm muscles relaxed, but on point of contact against the opponent's limb, tense it, blocking with forearm

e) X Block

Stand in fighting stance, hands on guard position, eyes on the opponent. Bend your knees, and keep the hip relaxed. As soon as the opponent strikes let both the hands move from the waist towards the opponent punch in a cross fashion or as the name denotes in a X formation. The block should be done as though pressing the opponent's punch towards the ceiling. Arm muscles relaxed, but on point of contact against the opponent's limb, tense it, blocking with forearm.

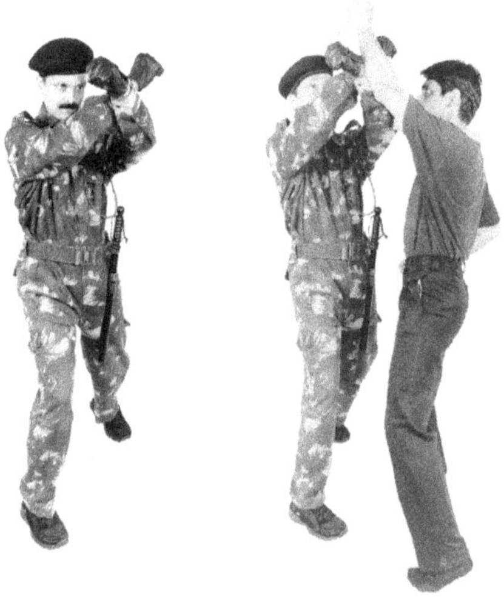

f) Inside Knee Block

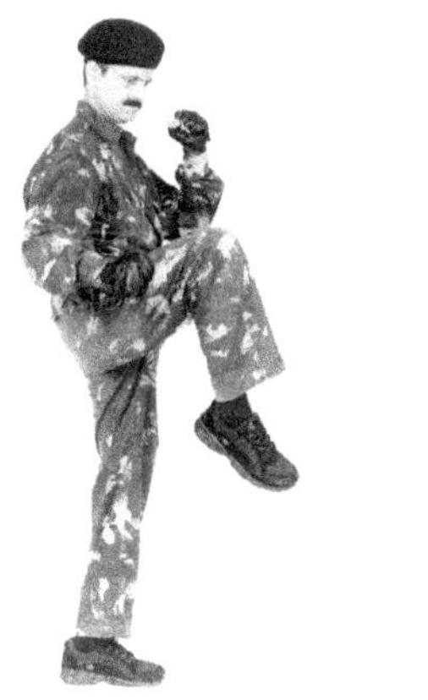 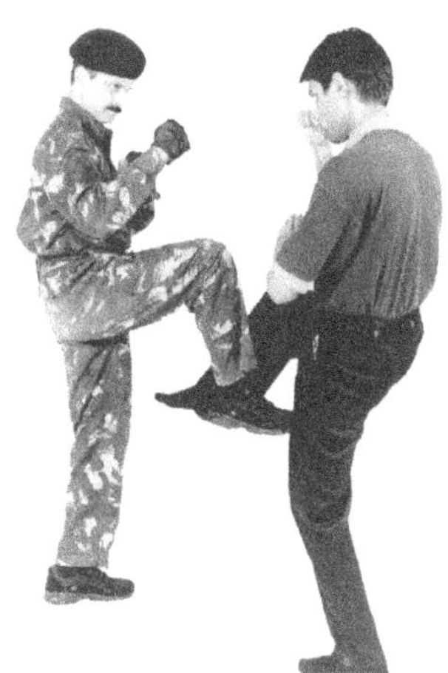

Stand in fighting stance, hands on guard position, eyes on the opponent. Bend your knees, and keep the hip relaxed. As soon as the opponent strikes let the leading leg travel up and across the stomach and groin region across the body towards the rear leg position. Body weight on the rear leg, with balanced maintained. Blocking is done with the inside part of the knee or shin bone. Knees bend, toes pointing towards the ground. Leading leg's thigh parallel towards the ground.

g) Outside Knee Block

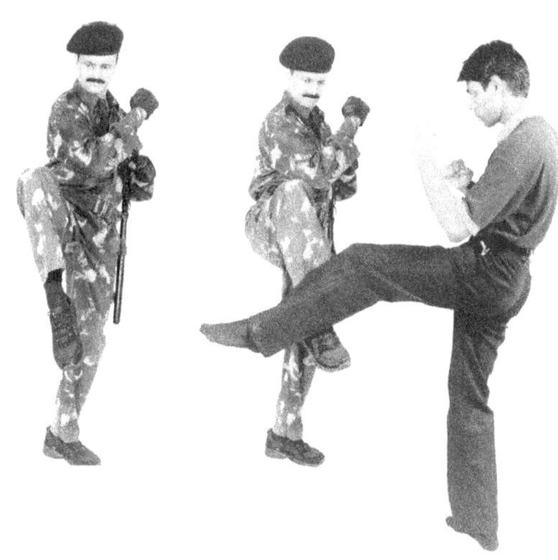

Stand in fighting stance, hands on guard position, eyes on the opponent. Bend your knees, and keep the hip relaxed. As soon as the opponent strikes let the leading leg travel from the rear leg position across the stomach and groin region across the body towards the outward position. Body weight on the rear leg, with balanced maintained. Blocking is done with the outside part of the knee or shin bone. Knees bend, toes pointing towards the ground. The leading leg's thigh is parallel towards the ground.

❑   ❑   ❑

This page intentionally left blank

Chapter 5
Footwork

Always give way to your opponents attack, while countering in the wake of his own movement and loss of balance.

Footwork

In our infancy we progressed through different stages. We crawled before walking, walked before running and ran before jumping, hopping or skipping. In the same way, one should learn to move from one stance to another in a smooth fluid motion, without breaking the rhythm and at the same time, do not lose balance. After some proficiency, we will be able to run through our stance or shuffle, hop, skip, and jump with ease. These stages will help us to gain or lessen distances between opponents, as well as give us a change of pace. Skill in footwork is very important in the art of fighting. It is heavily relied upon, in attack, defense, deception and conservation of energy. Without footwork, the fighter is like immobile cannon which cannot be directed at the enemy line. The speed and power of our punches and kicks depends on our nimble feet and balanced body.

I Stationery Stances:

Your stance has three functions. Firstly, it affects your breathing and consequently your mental framework (a well define posture, will give confidence and ample supply of oxygen for the flight and flee response, as mentioned in Chp.2). Secondly, it is the first positive move you will make in a violent situation. It shows that you have accepted the possibility of violence. Thirdly, it puts you in the best position to attack or counter-attack. A stance may also have the added advantage of deterring a would-be attacker. He may conclude that you know what you are doing, and half the battle is won, before the launch of any attack.

Fighting Stance:

Spread your leg about twice the shoulder width. Front leg bent and toes at an angle of 45⁰, knee making an obtuse angle. The rear leg toe touching the floor, heel raised up. Toe pointing to the front leg heel, as though both the front and rear legs are align to each other. Knee bent, but do not bend or lean towards the front leg, but move away from it. Groin pulled inside for protection. Weight on front leg 55% and rear leg 45%. Hip relaxed chest and back straight. Eyes looking straight ahead towards the opponent. The leading leg's hand straight in front of the body, elbow bent at right angle, fingers facing the sky. Forearm covers from the waist line to the nose. The leading leg and hand are in aligning towards each other. The rear leg's hand is bent at the elbow at an angle of 90⁰, fingers facing the opponent, forearm covering the solar plexus and the chest line. Body relaxed, no tensing of any muscles required.

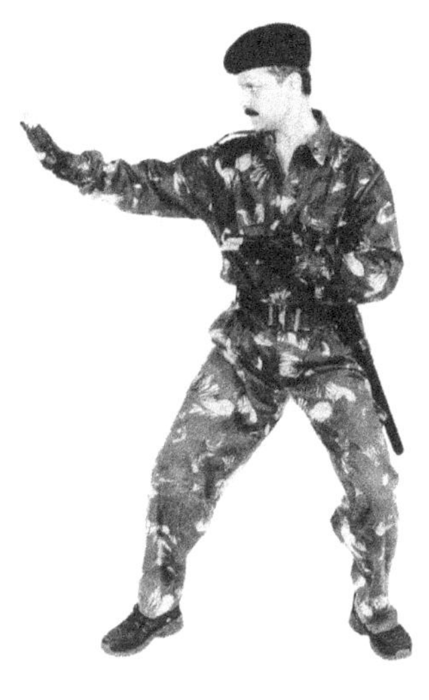

Archer Stance:

In this stance, the front leg is curved like a bow and the back leg is straight, extended like an arrow. When used with combination of the other stance, this strong posture will increase the range of your hands. Spread your legs apart about two and half the time of your shoulder distance. Point the toes of the front leg straight, whereas the toes of your rear leg will be at an angle of 45⁰, from the front to the side. Bend the knees of the front leg so the thigh is parallel to the floor. The knee and toe of your front foot should be aligned. Extend the rear leg fully. In this stance the front bent leg will be carrying 70% of the body weight whereas the rear leg will be carrying 30%. Hands on hip, eyes in front. Entire body relaxed.

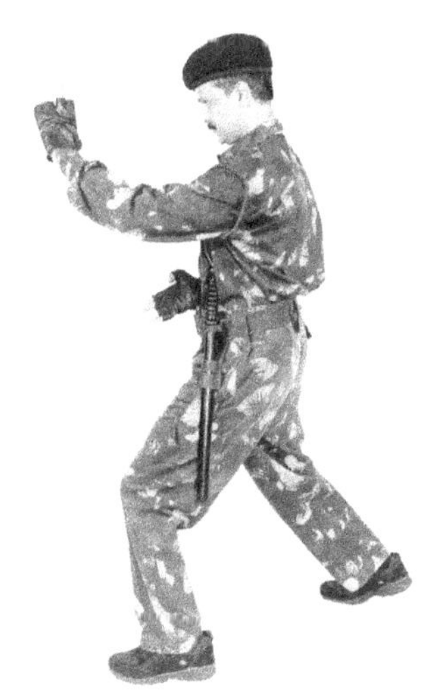

Free Stance (Cat Stance):

In this stance, assume a crouched position; the leg which is free is usually used for the purpose of kicking. This stance has a very good aspect for further mobility and counter attack positioning. Spread your legs same as the width of your shoulder. Point your rear foot outward and your front foot straight ahead. Align the toes of your front foot with the heel of your rear foot. Keep your back straight. Lower the body as though sitting in a chair. Rear thigh should be parallel to the floor. The heel of the front foot should be off the floor. The toes should be curled inwards, gripping the floor. Keep your body low so that very little of it is exposed to an attack. The tension and pain in the rear thigh will disappear once you are accustomed to the stance, 90% weight on rear leg and 10% on front leg.

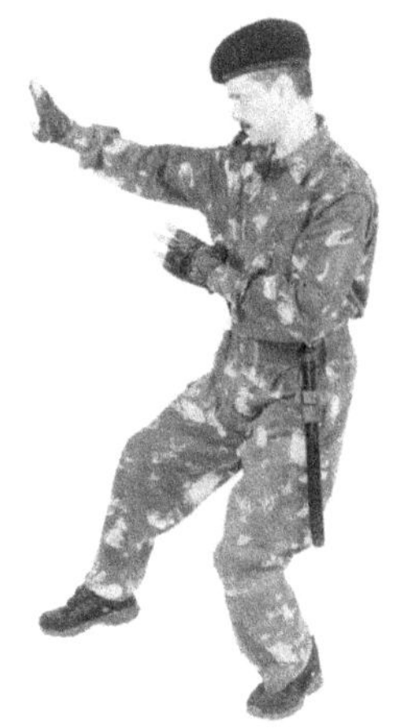

One Leg Stance (Crane Stance):

This stance is primarily used for attacking, by the help of kicks. Lift one leg up, until knee comes up to chest level. The other leg supports your entire body and the foot is flat on the floor pointing towards the front or at an angle of 45º. Bend the knee of the supporting foot, do not lock it. Point the raised leg toe towards the supporting leg keeping it slightly bent. Full body weight on supporting leg.

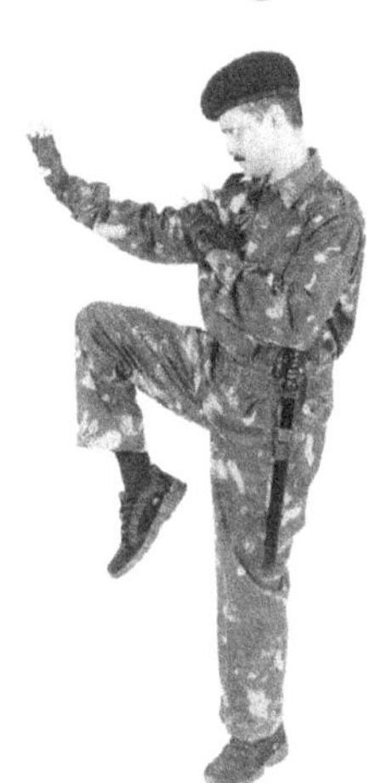

Horse stance (Crane Stance):

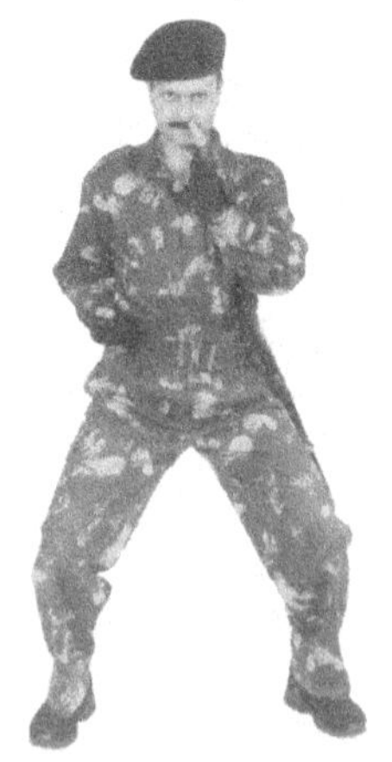

As indicated, this stance derives its name from the squatting position of a horse rider. It is a common stance for all martial arts. In the initial stages, you will experience leg pains, but once you strengthen your legs the pain will disappear. Spread your legs apart, about twice the width of your shoulders, toes pointing at angle of 45º. Squat down as if you are sitting on a horse, with your knees apart. One hand on hip, while the other hands in front as shown in the accompanying figure. Back should be straight and knees slightly bent. Body weight distributed equally on both the legs. Focus both mind and strength towards lower abdominal region.

II Moving Footwork:

In everyday life one does not pay a lot of attention to how one move around. Roads and paths are flat or well lit. In a self defense situation, however, how you move may be of crucial importance. When you are under stress and concentrating on an assailant, moving around may be difficult. There is a great danger that you may move haphazardly, even after learning all the attacking and defending moves, you will be like immovable cannon. So practice all your attacking and defending techniques while moving forward, backward, sideward or to launch the final assault then in hopping footwork. Practice all the move till you can glide through your movement without any major effort.

Forward or Backward Move:

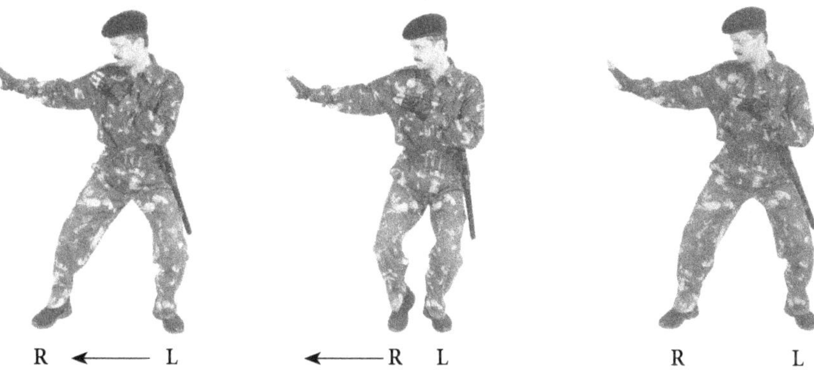

This foot work is very important to close on your opponent to attack or back out while blocking. It is a small series of steps taken in front or back at speed. From fighting stance, proceed forward, first take a step with the left leg and then step up with the right leg and keep on advancing this way towards the opponent. Remember this footwork has to be done in speed.

Note: To retreat, use the same principle i.e. take a step with the right leg towards the back, then pull the left leg towards the right leg and so on. The retreat technique is useful for defending, whereas the forward shuffle technique is useful for attacking.

Sideways Move (Side step to Right):

While facing the opponent, from fighting stance take a step to the right side with the help of right leg and then pull the left leg towards the right side. All movements should be done smoothly and gracefully in one smooth motion and with speed.

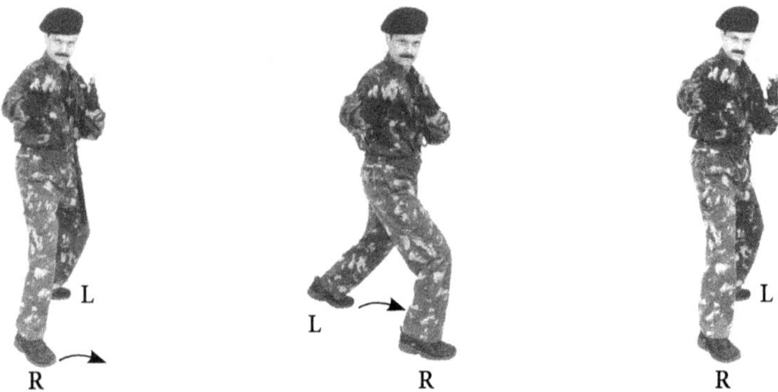

Sideways Move (Side step to Left):

From fighting stance take a step towards the left side, (with the left leg) and then pull the right leg towards the left side. All movements should be done smoothly and gracefully in one smooth motion and with speed. Remember to face the opponent and be ready to counter any moves he/she makes.

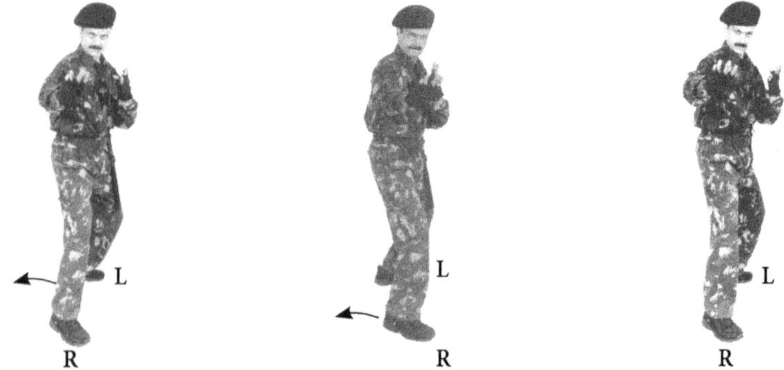

Note: Remember footwork has to be learned like any other skill, if you don't, then your movements will be clumsy. Once you learn it, you will be master of deceit, especially when moving forward, backward and sideward.

Chapter 6

Basic Attacks

Make your opponent defeat himself.

Basic Attacks

Man has never been able to know what the potential of his mind and body is. Proper training in Martial Arts and particularly Chi Kung/Qigong (Pranayam) can help him to know himself. When a practitioner trains in the use of external weapons (e.g. stick, sword, spear, chain, etc.) for self defense, then he is underestimating his own natural weapons, which are far more superior than the above, and once a practitioner underestimates or ignores his own natural weapons then he can never develop and use them effectively. So a serious practitioner of Self Defense should first concentrate in developing his own natural weapons.

How to hold a Fist:

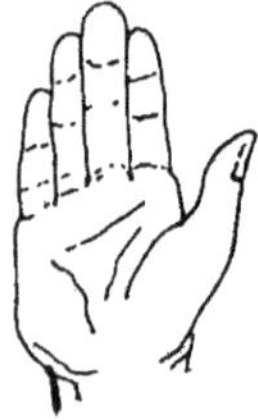

Open Palm

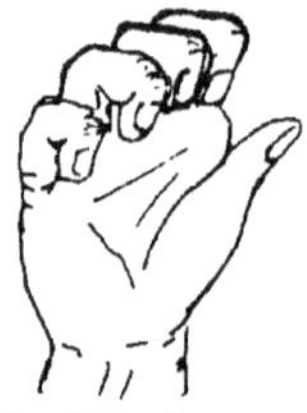

Bend the first two phalanges of all the fingers

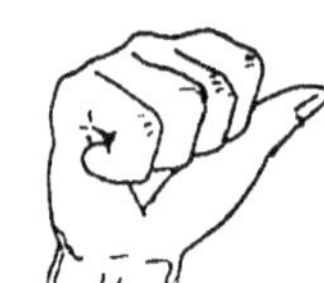

Bend the third phalanges of all fingers towards palm

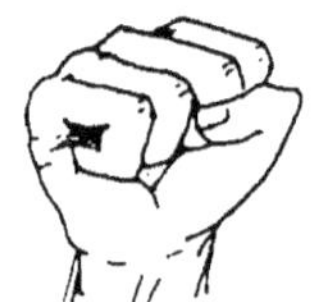

Now clench the fist tight & place thumb on first 2 fingers

Points for punching:

1. The power of a punch comes from the hips and shoulders, not the arm. The arm only transmits the power. Learn to punch using the hips and shoulders.

2. Before actually striking, keep the arm and fist relaxed. A tense arm cannot move fast. On impact, clench the fist tightly and rotate (cork-screw) it round so that the palm faces down (straight punches).

3. Punch through the target.

4. Hit with the first two big knuckles of the hand i.e. knuckle of the index and middle finger. Keep the thumb tucked out of the way, touching the index and middle finger between the first and second joints. On impact your knuckles, wrist and elbows should form a straight line.

5. Punch when advancing or stationery, not when moving backwards.

6. A straight punch is faster than a hooked one, but a hooked one is very powerful and swings in from outside the line of vision.

7. Double up your punches, either head and body or right and left. Do not expect that one punch will do the trick. Put in a volley of punches and backup with a powerful hook punch.

1) Punch:

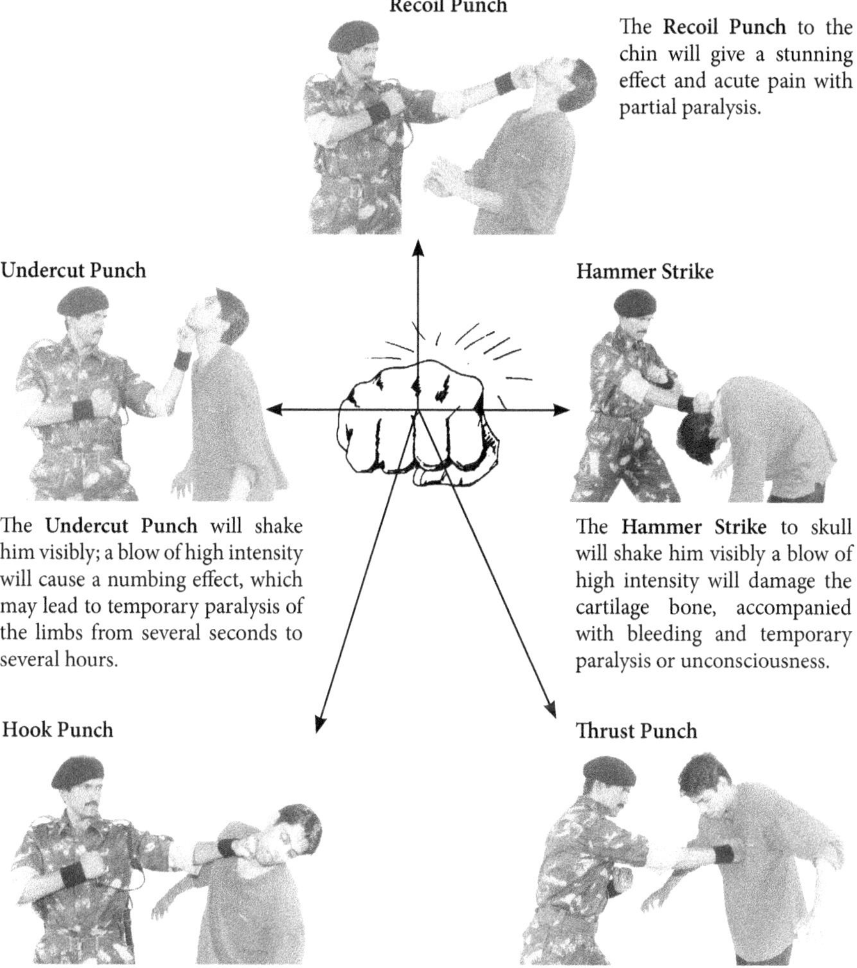

Recoil Punch

The **Recoil Punch** to the chin will give a stunning effect and acute pain with partial paralysis.

Undercut Punch

The **Undercut Punch** will shake him visibly; a blow of high intensity will cause a numbing effect, which may lead to temporary paralysis of the limbs from several seconds to several hours.

Hammer Strike

The **Hammer Strike** to skull will shake him visibly a blow of high intensity will damage the cartilage bone, accompanied with bleeding and temporary paralysis or unconsciousness.

Hook Punch

The **Hook punch** to the neck will shake him visibly; a blow of high intensity will damage the windpipe, accompanied with bleeding and temporary paralysis or unconscious.

Thrust Punch

The **Thrust Punch** to the solar plexus with a blow of high intensity will cause internal haemorrhage and maybe death.

2) Open Palm:

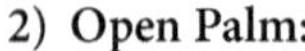

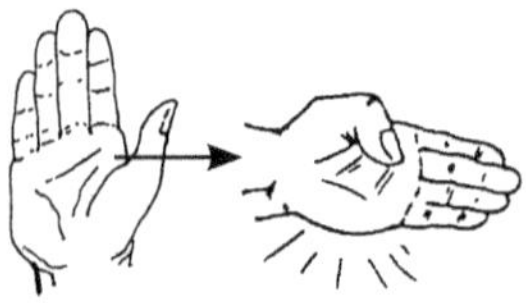

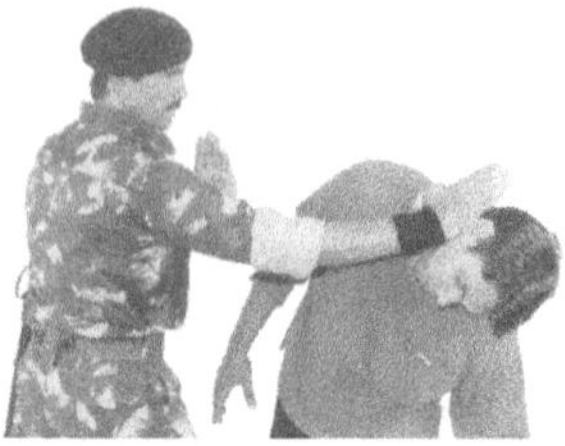

The **Chop** to the side of the neck will shake him visibly with temporary paralysis, whereas a blow of high intensity will cause internal hemorrhage and sometime a choking sensation, which may lead to a state of unconscious.

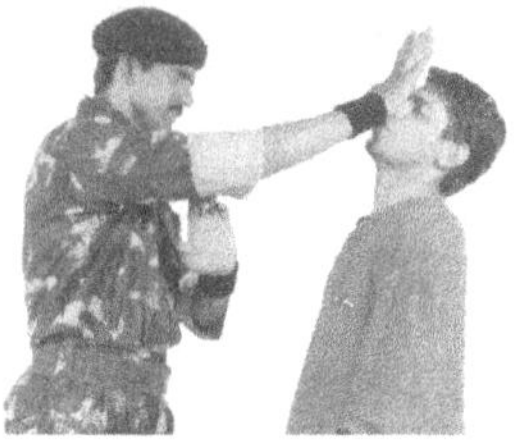

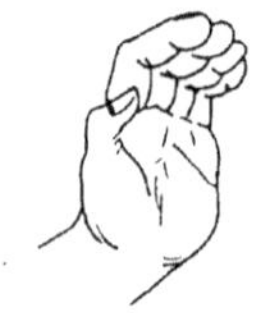

The **Bear's paw** strike to the nose may lead to severe damage of the nose.

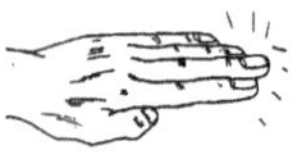

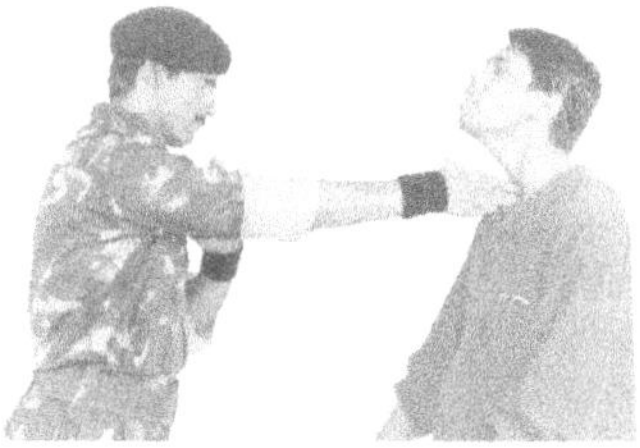

The **Finger stab strike** to neck may lead to choking and temporary paralysis which could be fatal.

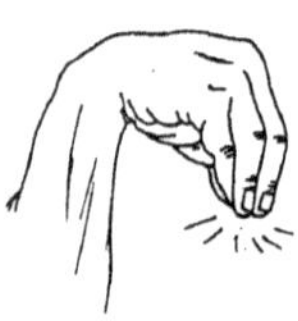

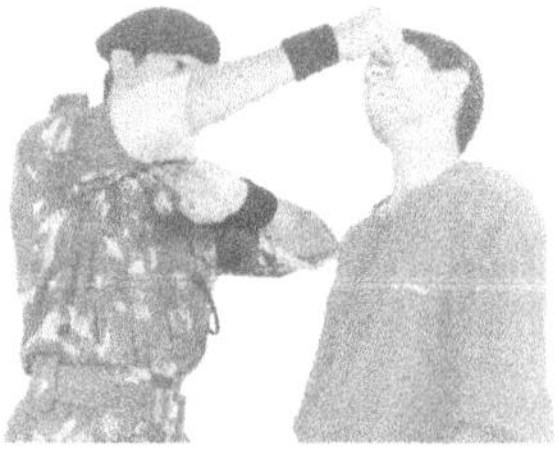

A **beak strike** to the eye may lead to permanent blindness.

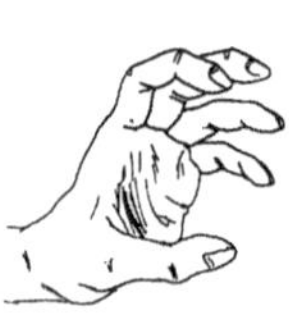

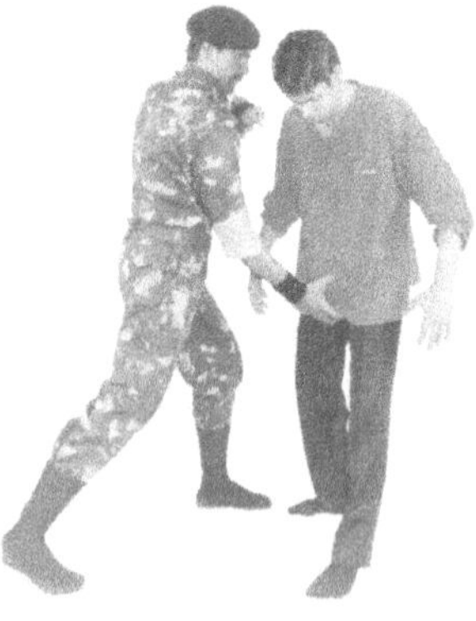

A **Tiger Claw** the groin will lead to temporary paralysis or a state of unconsciousness for hours.

3) Elbow Strike:

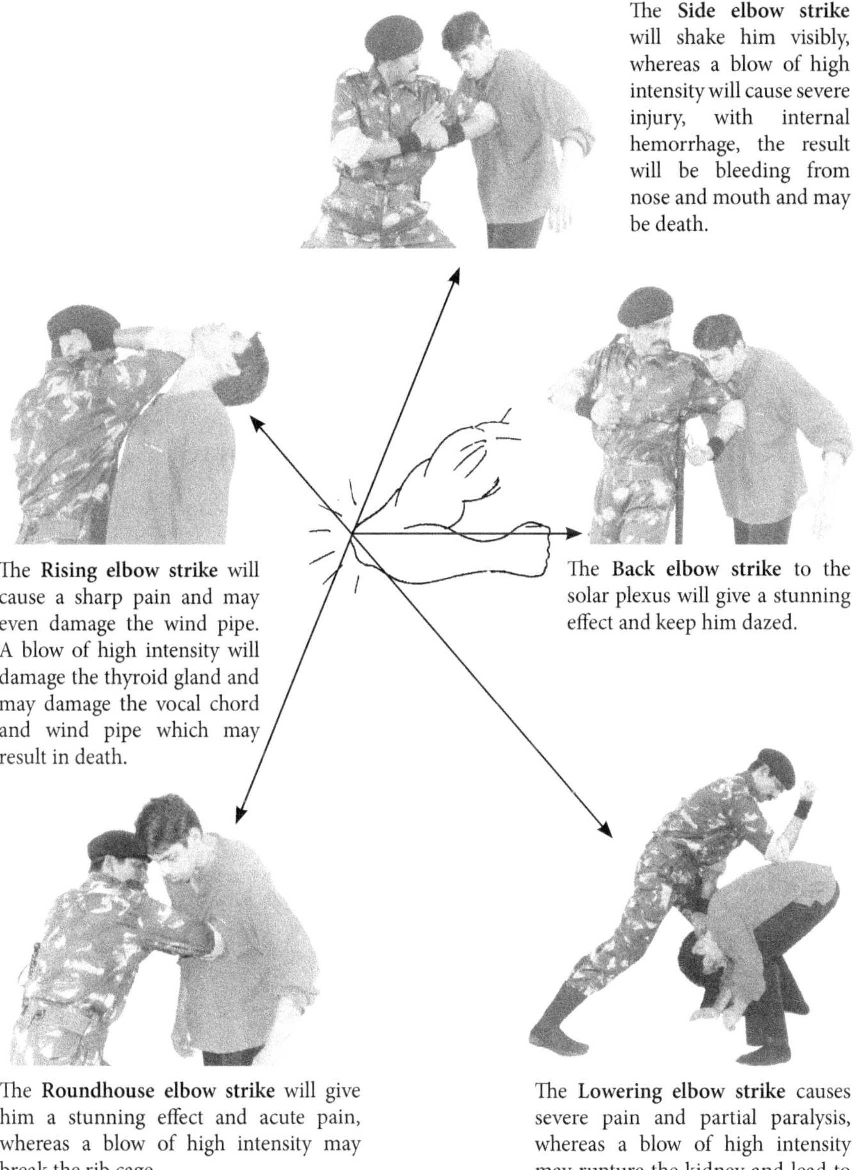

The **Side elbow strike** will shake him visibly, whereas a blow of high intensity will cause severe injury, with internal hemorrhage, the result will be bleeding from nose and mouth and may be death.

The **Rising elbow strike** will cause a sharp pain and may even damage the wind pipe. A blow of high intensity will damage the thyroid gland and may damage the vocal chord and wind pipe which may result in death.

The **Back elbow strike** to the solar plexus will give a stunning effect and keep him dazed.

The **Roundhouse elbow strike** will give him a stunning effect and acute pain, whereas a blow of high intensity may break the rib cage.

The **Lowering elbow strike** causes severe pain and partial paralysis, whereas a blow of high intensity may rupture the kidney and lead to complications which may result in death.

Points for Kicking:

1.   Raise the knee, as if stepping up on to a high box, flick the foot out (side, back or front) and pull it quickly back – the movement in one continuous whole.

2.   Stand straight, do not protrude the hips back.

3.   If wearing shoes, as you will be in most self-defense situations, kick with the toe-cap, but make your foot and ankle firm. Aim to connect with a particular part of your shoe or foot if you kick in any other manner.

4.   For kicks higher than the groin, you will need to loosen up your ham-strings and hips. The lower you kick the quicker and faster it will be.

4) Knee Strike:

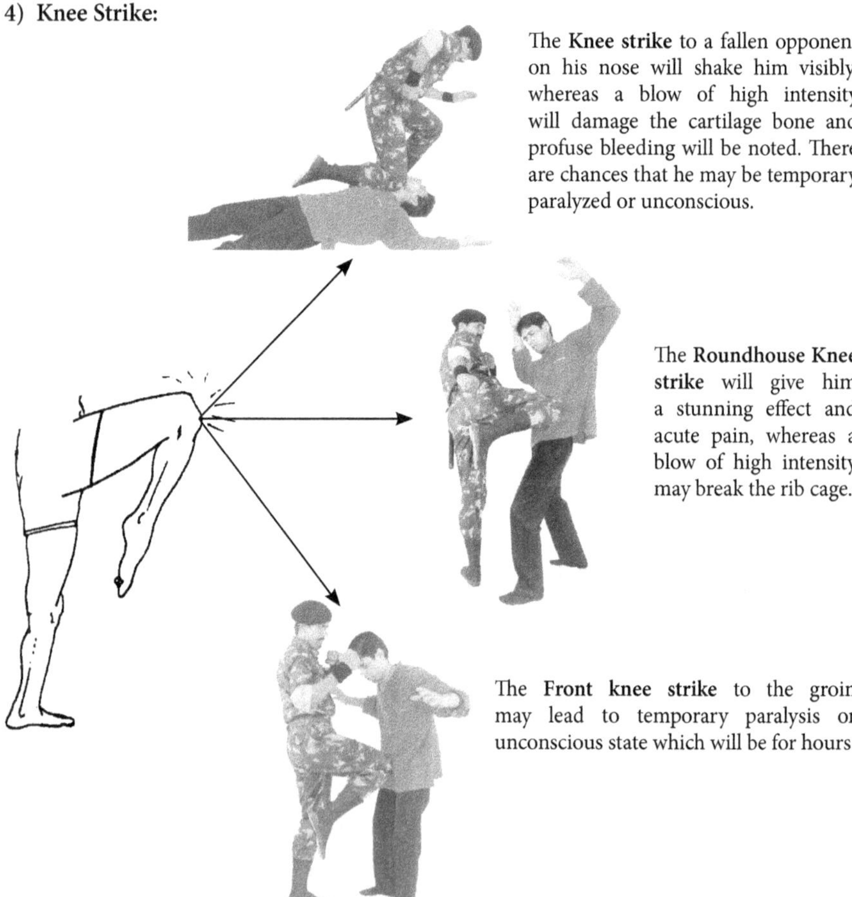

The **Knee strike** to a fallen opponent on his nose will shake him visibly, whereas a blow of high intensity will damage the cartilage bone and profuse bleeding will be noted. There are chances that he may be temporary paralyzed or unconscious.

The **Roundhouse Knee strike** will give him a stunning effect and acute pain, whereas a blow of high intensity may break the rib cage.

The **Front knee strike** to the groin may lead to temporary paralysis or unconscious state which will be for hours.

5) Feet Strike:

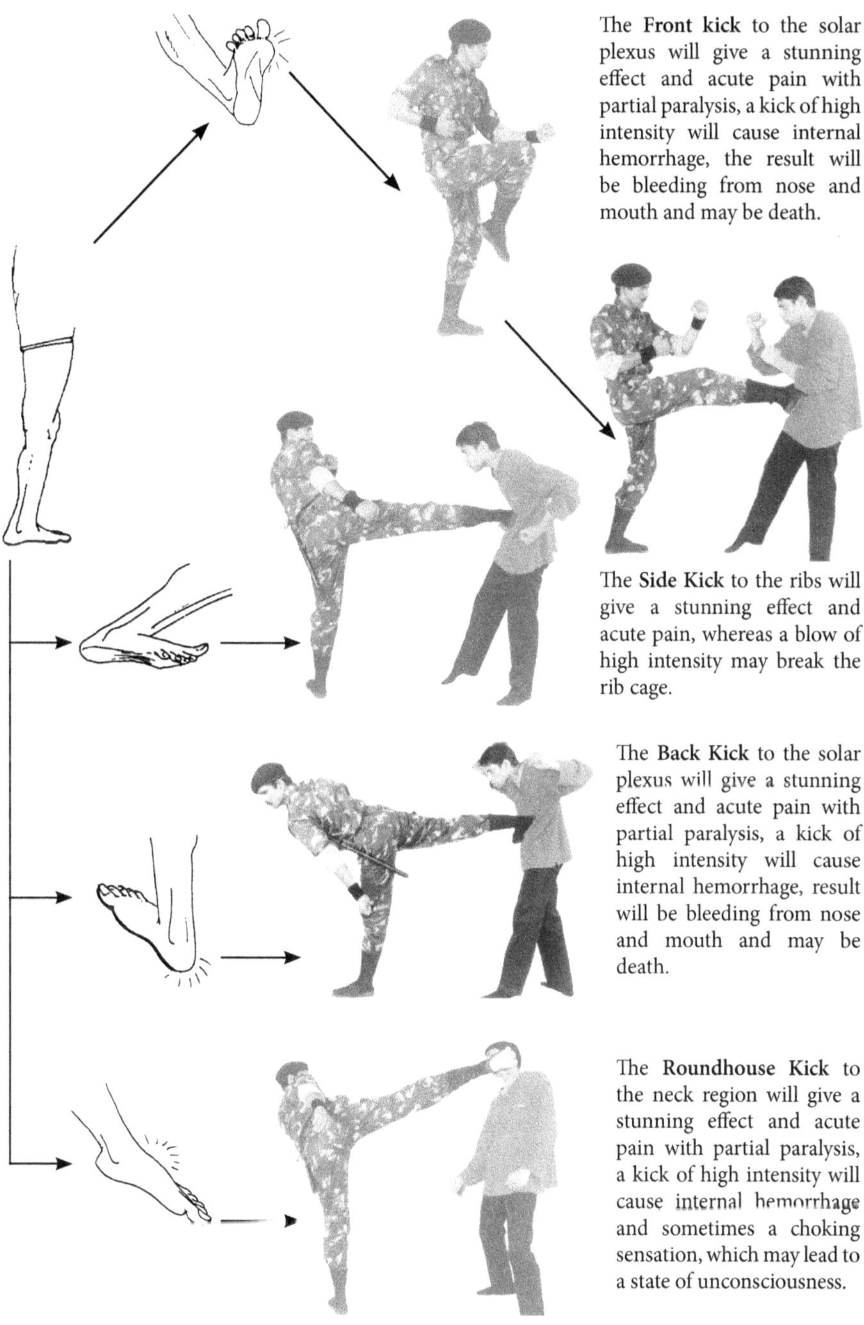

The **Front kick** to the solar plexus will give a stunning effect and acute pain with partial paralysis, a kick of high intensity will cause internal hemorrhage, the result will be bleeding from nose and mouth and may be death.

The **Side Kick** to the ribs will give a stunning effect and acute pain, whereas a blow of high intensity may break the rib cage.

The **Back Kick** to the solar plexus will give a stunning effect and acute pain with partial paralysis, a kick of high intensity will cause internal hemorrhage, result will be bleeding from nose and mouth and may be death.

The **Roundhouse Kick** to the neck region will give a stunning effect and acute pain with partial paralysis, a kick of high intensity will cause internal hemorrhage and sometimes a choking sensation, which may lead to a state of unconsciousness.

Note:

1. All natural weapons should be practiced to both the sides to have fluency in movement.

2. These are some of the variations you can practice but with little effort, you can develop your own variation.

3. For all kicking techniques balance is very important, don't sacrifice balance for reach, since you will lose power and the technique may become weak.

4. Toughen the natural weapons either by striking a bag of grains or a soft mattress, then graduate to punching bag filled with sand or the telephone directory, this will condition and toughen your natural weapon.

5. All strikes which lead to severe injury, possible permanent injury or possible death - these types or the degree of punishment is justified only in the face of vicious, deadly attack where your life is in real danger.

❑   ❑   ❑

Chapter 7
Unarmed Techniques

Try to defeat your opponent the instant he attacks you.

Unarmed Techniques

Ability in some form of self-defense is becoming more and more necessary in today's modern world, for the simple fact that violence is on the increase. There seems to be no sign of any reversal in the continual annual increase in criminal activities. It is not practical to rely on the law enforcers to help you out, you have to act on your own. Knowledge of self-defense situation should convince you of the need for awareness, with knowledge and awareness you have achieved two-thirds of the way. If more people become adept at self-defense and are prepared then violence at all levels would surely decrease.

There are three aspects of self defense ability; KNOWLEDGE of the situation, AWARENESS and the actual physical ABILITY to deal with an attack. While speed is undoubtedly an essential factor in actual combat, a more important factor is OPPORTUNITY, which can only be seized through a correct judgment of the enemy's movements and a correct evaluation of his intentions. The toughest, most ferocious and skillful fighter can be beaten if he is day dreaming or not paying attention. Especially during night times, be aware of dark corners or doorway, or who is following you, by being aware you can take appropriate action. With some idea of self-defense situation and awareness, you will have already gained the first step in self-defense.

Often in the self-defense situation an attacker will catch hold of you, either to force you to do something, or to steady you prior to making a blow. The ways you can be caught can be divided roughly into three groups, wrist grabs, frontal holds, and rear holds. One point to note is in any grappling attack, one must be well balanced and have enough strength to surprised the opponent's strength and body weight with simple and effective techniques as given below. The next stage is to practice the actual techniques.

Techniques 1:

1.   The attacker is armed with a knife, and is
ready to lunge it into your abdominal region, you
are supposed to check his advances, with your eye
movement on his knife without provoking him.

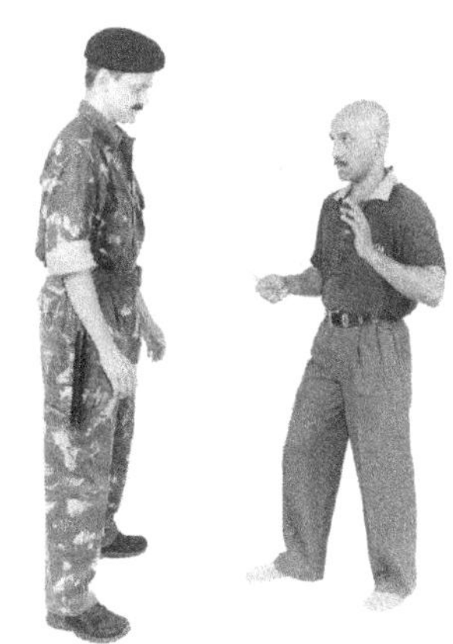

2.   The moment he charges in, step in front
with your left foot and control his striking hand
with your right hand, while the left hand is at your
left flank ready for action.

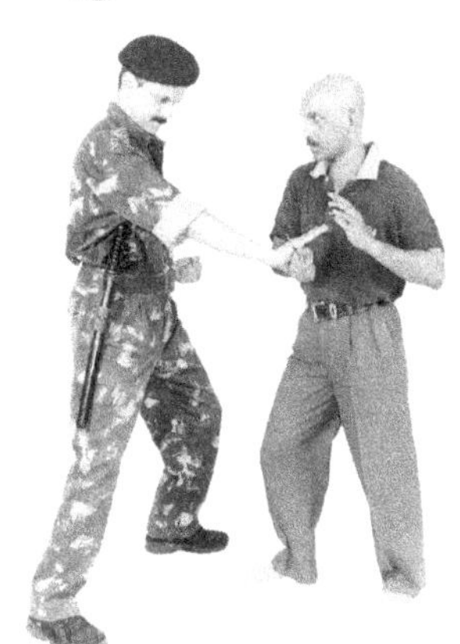

3.   Then twist your body weight on to your
right leg and simultaneously grab his attacking
hand with your right hand at the wrist and twist
it downward, simultaneously with your left hand
strike with your forearms on his elbow joints to
make his grip weak. Continue applying pressure
with your left hand downward and apply pressure
upward with your right hand.

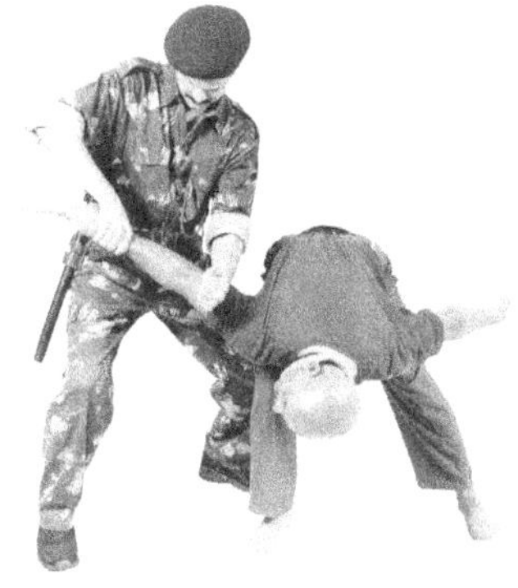

Note: If all these movements are done in one quick succession, then there is a possibility of snapping his elbow.

Techniques 2:

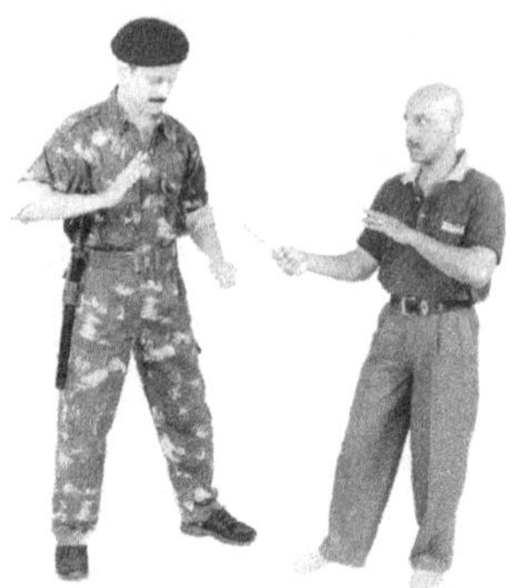

◄   1.   The attacker is armed with a knife, and is ready to lunge it into your abdominal region, you are supposed to check his advances, with your eye movement on his knife without provoking him.

2.   The moment he charges in, step in front ►
with your left foot and control his striking hand with your right hand, by holding his wrist tightly, while the left hand strikes with a chop attack into his crook of the elbows, this will give him a jerk, by which he may be off balance.

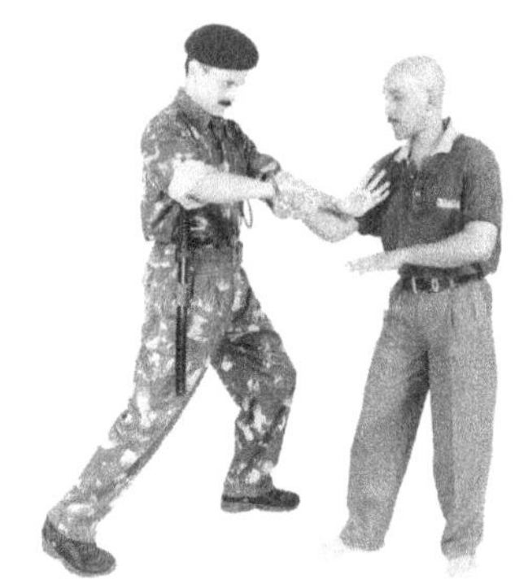

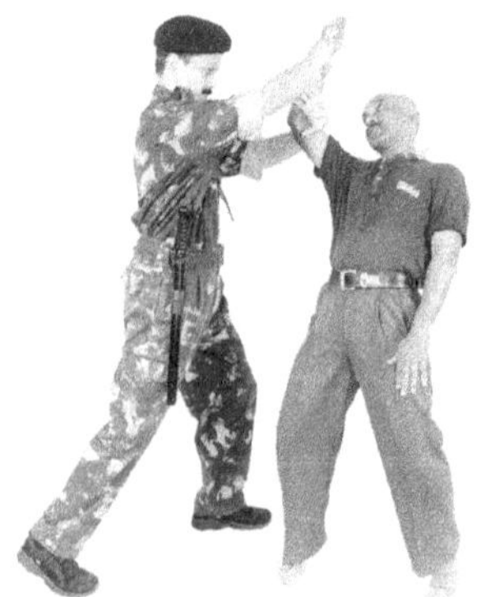

◄   3.   Then twist your body and transfer body weight on your left leg and simultaneously lift his weapon hand, by your rear hand (right hand), without loosening your grip, open your palm and rotate it towards the little finger side and hold his wrist tight, while the left hand will slip in and tries to hold your wrist. This motion will weaken his balance, & he may loose ground.

4.   Continue applying pressure with your ►
right hand, by stepping in front with your right foot to his rear right. Your right thighs will be behind his right thigh, the continuity of the pressure by your right hand will trip him over your thighs and he will loose his balance and crash on the ground, where you can follow up with any of the finishing techniques as shown in the attacking chapter.

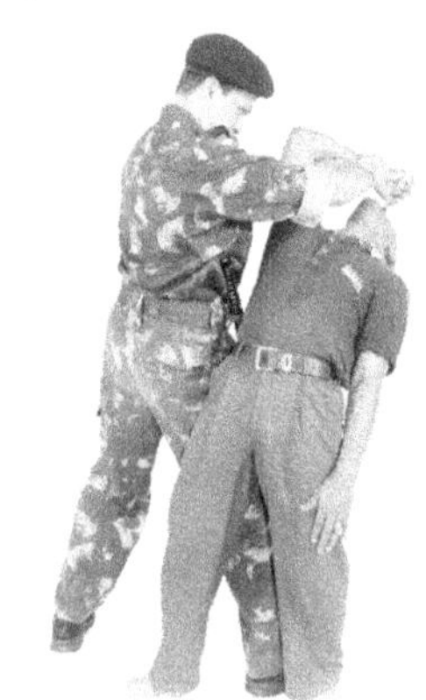

Techniques 3:

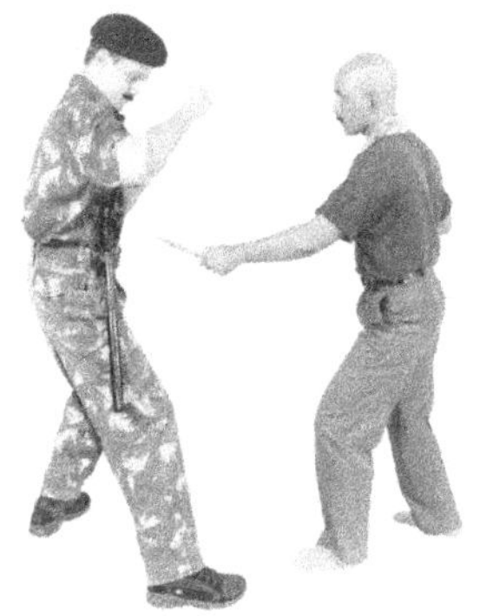

◁   1.   The attacker is armed with a knife, and is ready to lunge it into your abdominal region, you are supposed to check his advances, with your eye movement on his knife without provoking him. Pull in your abdomen region if the knife comes near your body and keep your hands in on guard position, ready to defend yourself.

2.   Hold his attacking wrist with your leading hand, so as your thumb is on top of his back palm, body weight still on the back foot. Control his weapon by the wrist, and see that the knife is pointing away from you.   ▷

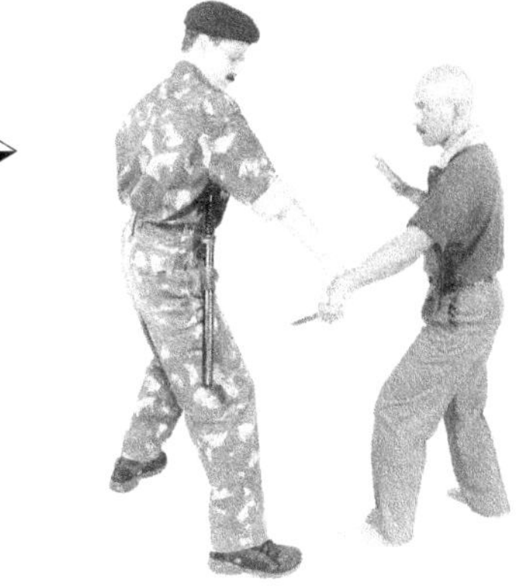

◁   3.   Rotate your leading hand, by holding the opponent's hand and turning it clockwise, with the help of your rear hand, simultaneously apply pressure with your thumb on the back of his palm, this will create tremendous pain and he will loose balance.

4.   Immediately step forward with the rear leg (left leg) next to his leading leg, this will create a circular motion, by twisting your hip clockwise, and creating a sort of vortex, where he is trapped, and looses his balance over your leading leg (left leg) thighs. Continue your hands and wrist pressure to the inner side of the vortex, which will imbalance him and he will be open to any counter attacks.   ▷

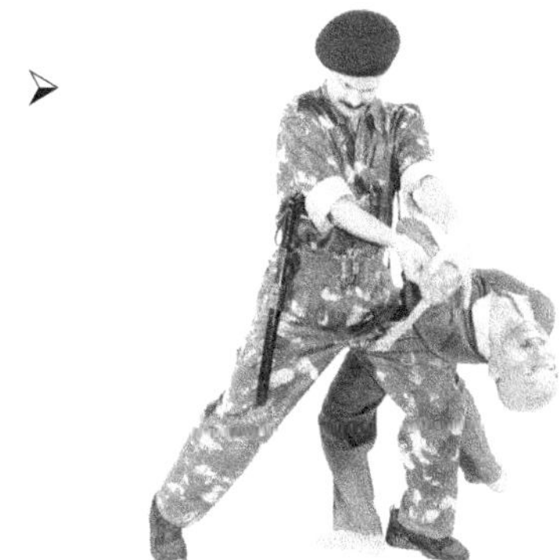

Techniques 4:

1.   Your opponent's throw a punch at you
with his leading hand at face level. Immediately
transfer your body weight on the back leg, and be
ready to do an outside block with your rear hand
(left hand). Keep the other hand extended so as to
guard your open right flank region.

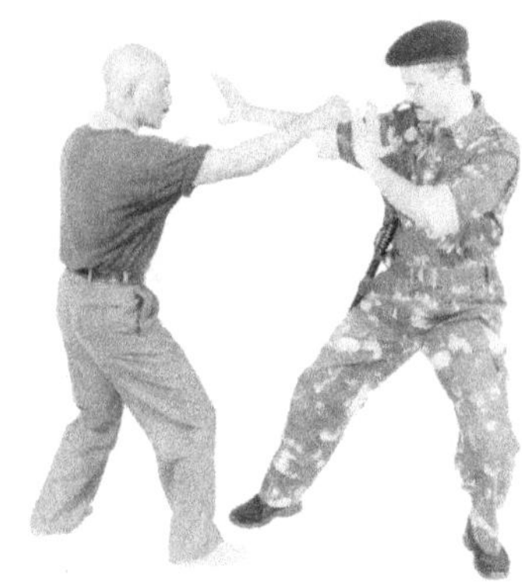

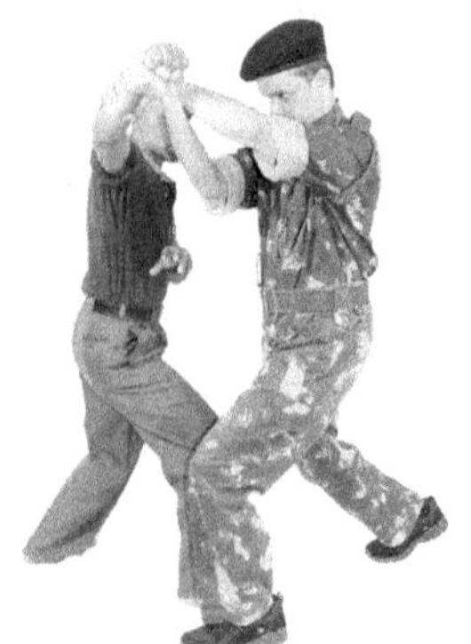

2.   Step forward with your rear leg (left
leg) to his extreme right; simultaneously hold his
punching hand with both your hands.

3.   Now   duck   your   body   under   the
opponent's right hand, and move in front with
the help of your right leg, both your hand is still
gripping the opponent's right hand and his hand
is over your shoulder, this move will twist his arm,
and he will be guided to move ahead.

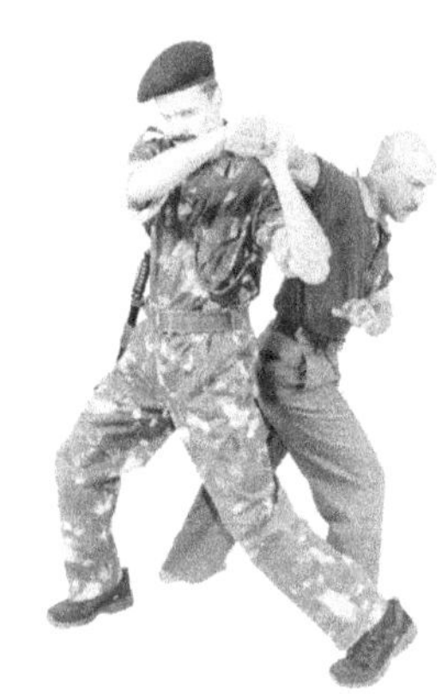

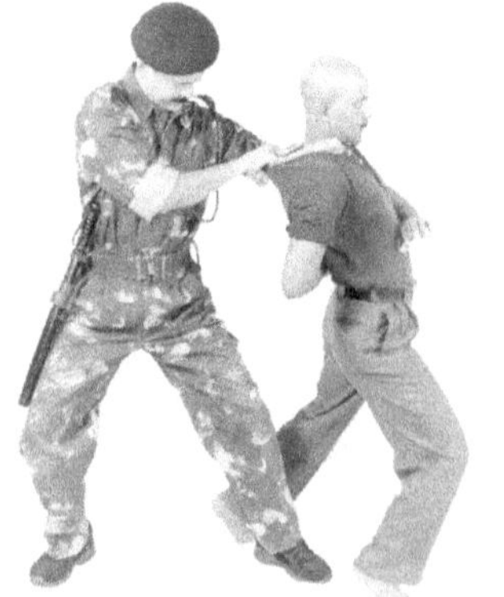

4.   Pull your left leg exactly behind him,
transfer your body weight on the back leg (right
leg). Simultaneously bring his seized hand behind
his back by pulling it with your left hand and hold
his collar with your right hand and drag him down,
automatically he will loose his balance and fall.

Techniques 5:

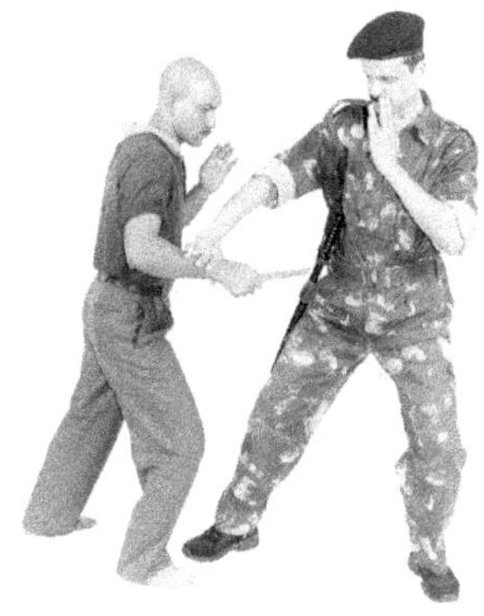

1.   The attacker is armed with a knife, and is already charging towards your midsection of your body, you are supposed to check his advances, by transferring your body weight on the back leg, this will create enough space to defend your midsection region. Then seize his attacking hand with your leading hand (right hand) on to his wrist, and keep your left hand in on guard position, ready to defend yourself.

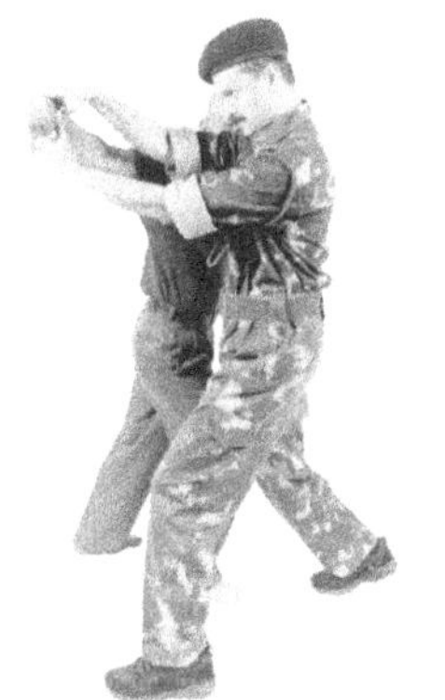

2.   Then step in front with the rear leg (left leg), hold on to the opponent's wrist with the left hand and left thumb on the back of his palm, and shift the right hand thumb on to the back of his palm.

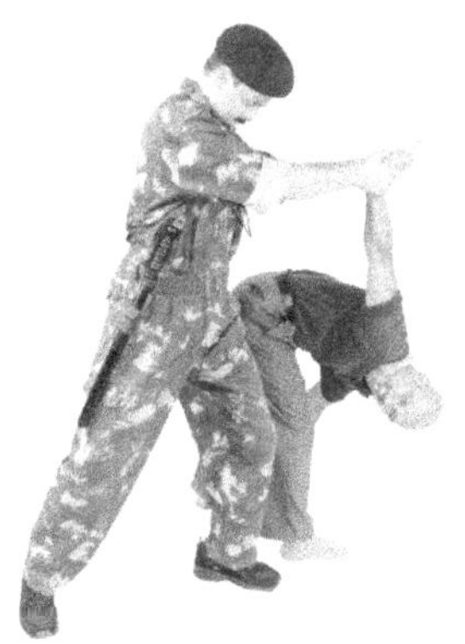

3.   Immediately turn around with your right leg rotating your body keeping the left leg as an axis's. Simultaneously keep on building pressure on the opponent's wrist, with both your hand, this will give intense pain to your opponent, and he will loose his grip on the knife.

Techniques 6:

1.   The attacker charges in front and holds your belt in a very threatening manner with his right hand. Be steady and maintain your balance on both your feet. Also check his advances, by keeping an eye over him without provoking him. Pull in your abdomen if the grip is too tight near your waist and keep your hands in on guard position, ready to defend yourself.

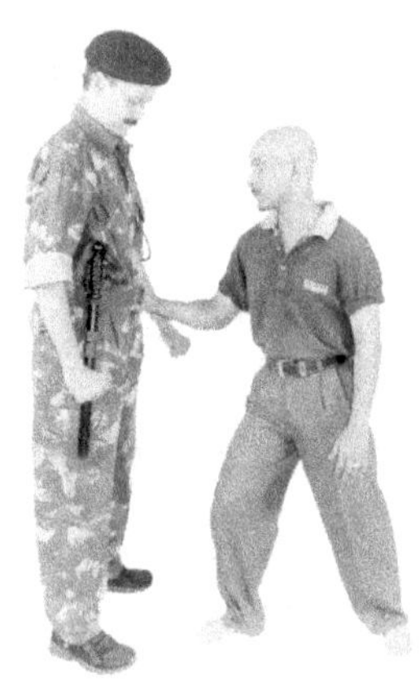

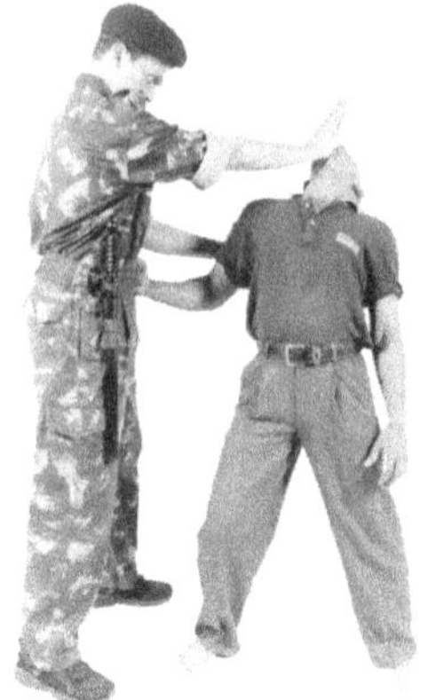

2.   Hold his right hand with your left hand and strike with the open palm to his nose region, this will visibly shake him and loosen his grip on your belt region.

3.   Immediately on loosening of his grip, grab his right wrist with your right hand, and then strike with your forearm on his back of elbow, this will force the opponent to lean in front.

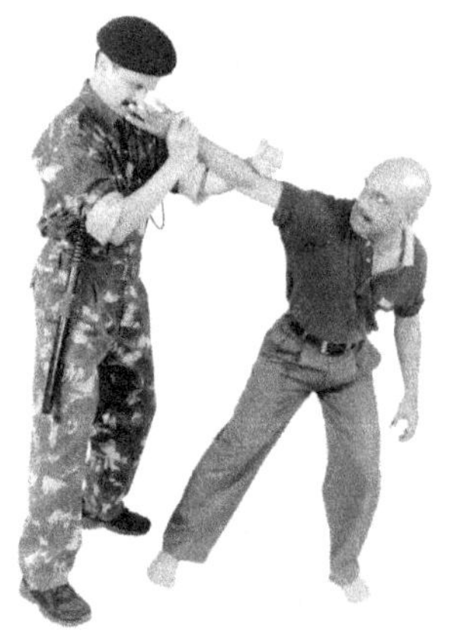

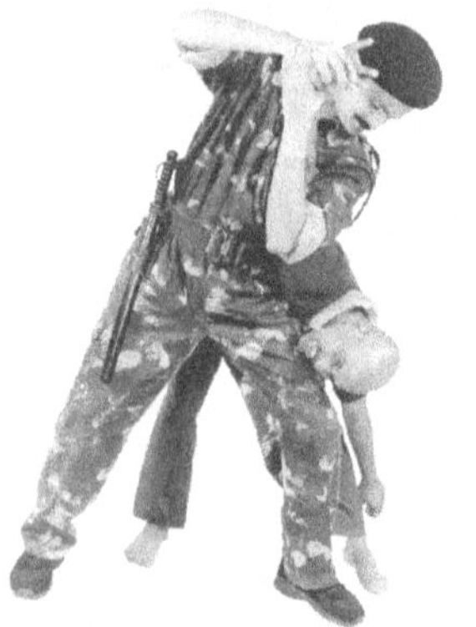

4.   Step with your left leg towards his rear leg, then slip your left hand around his elbow, by locking his right elbow stiff, and slip your right hand on to his wrist and bent in front, this will force him to bend down, then you can follow up with any counter attack techniques.

Techniques 7:

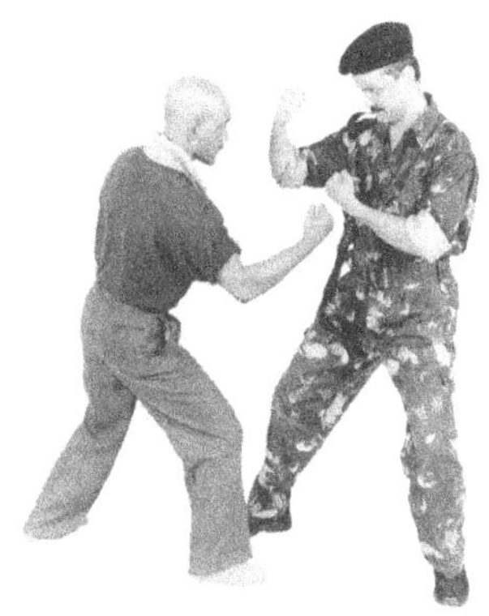

◁   1. Your opponent's is on the verge of throwing a punch with his leading hand to your face level. Immediately transfer your body weight on the back leg, and be ready to block with your rear hand (right hand). Keep the other hand extended so as to guard your left flank region.

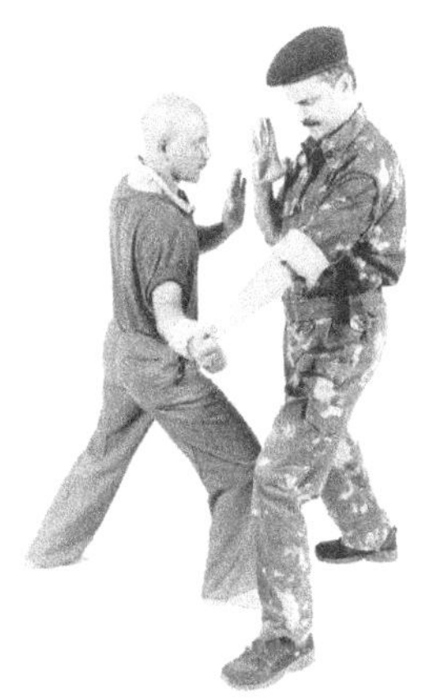

◁   2. Before he could move in more, step in front with your left leg and hold his right wrist with your left hand and keep your right hand to guard your right side of the flank.

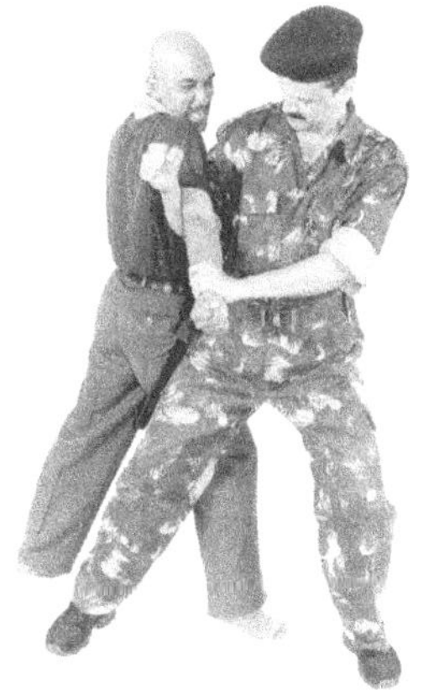

◁   3. Then step with your right foot in such a manner that you are exactly behind him and then slowly slip your right hand under his right arm into the crook of your elbow; this will jam his right elbow. Simultaneously apply pressure with your left hand downward, this will build intense pain and the opponent will be loosening his balance, then follow up with any of the counter attack techniques.

Techniques 8:

1.   Your opponent's throw a punch with his 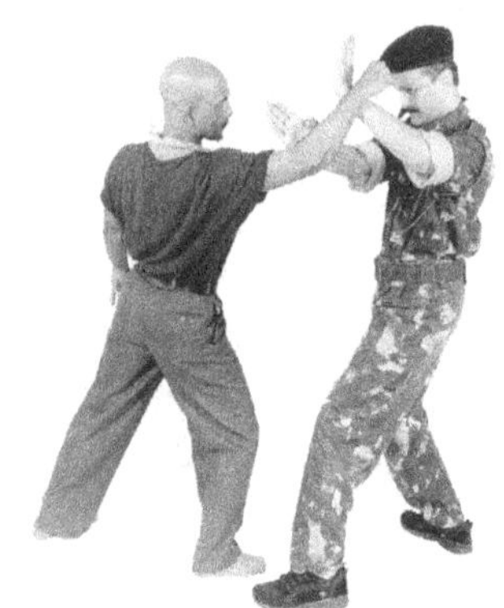 leading hand to your face level. Immediately transfer your body weight on the back leg, and do an outside block with your leading hand (left hand). With the other hand strike a chop into the crook of his elbow this will weaken his striking arm.

2.   Immediately hold the wrist of his striking 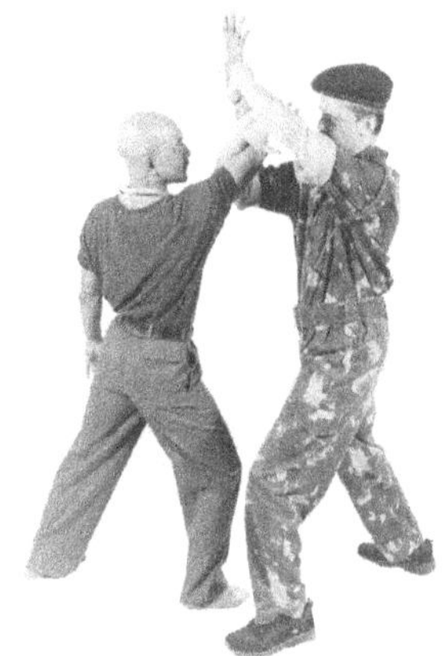 hand with your left hand and slip your right hand on to his elbow and try to hold your left hand with your right hand.

3.   Now step in front with your rear foot (right 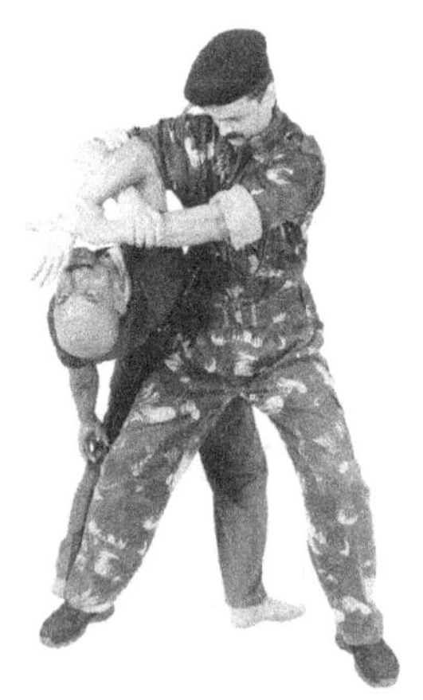 foot), you will be exactly behind him, continue the pressure of your hand and pull him down, this will give him intense pain and he will loose balance, follow up with any of the counter attack techniques to finish of your defense.

Techniques 9:

1. Your attacker tries to push you over with both his hand pressing on to your chest region, maintain a steady position by transferring your body weight on to the front leg, and keep your hand on guard position.

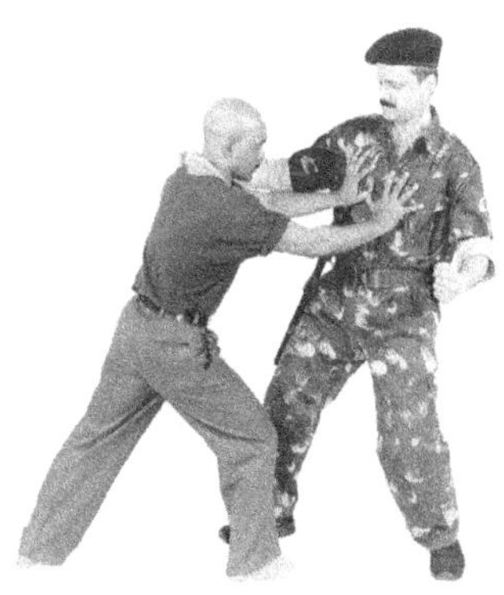

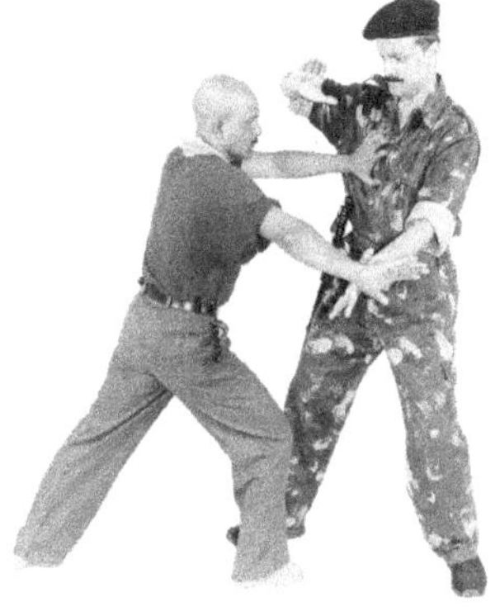

2. Slip your rear hand (left hand) under his right hand with a jerk and try to hold his wrist, simultaneously slightly turn your body towards your left side, this will ease the pressure of the push. Lift your right hand as to feign a chop strike to any part of his body; this will create a sort of confusion in the opponent.

3. Step forward with your rear foot (left foot), and lift the opponent's wrist with your left hand and press his shoulder region with your right hand, this will put your opponent off balance and he will be vulnerable to any attack.

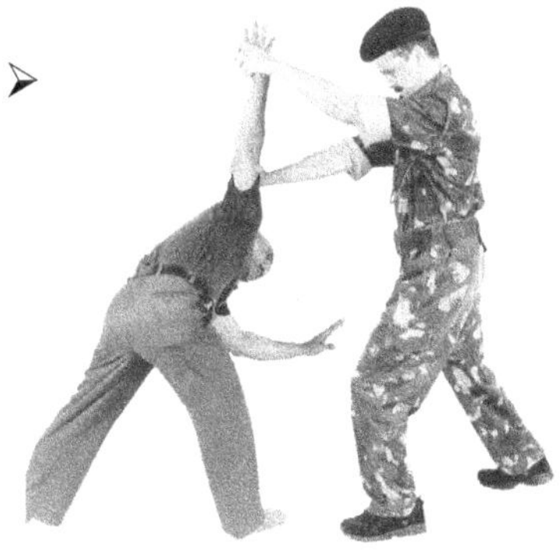

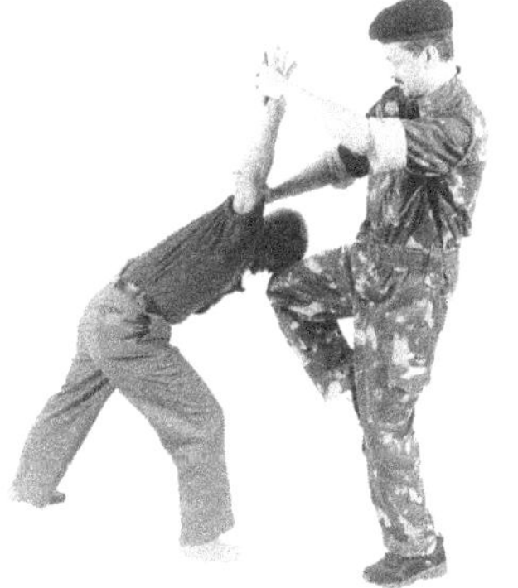

4. Then follow up with a knee strike to the opponent's face with the rear leg (right leg), this will give him crippling pain.

Techniques 10:

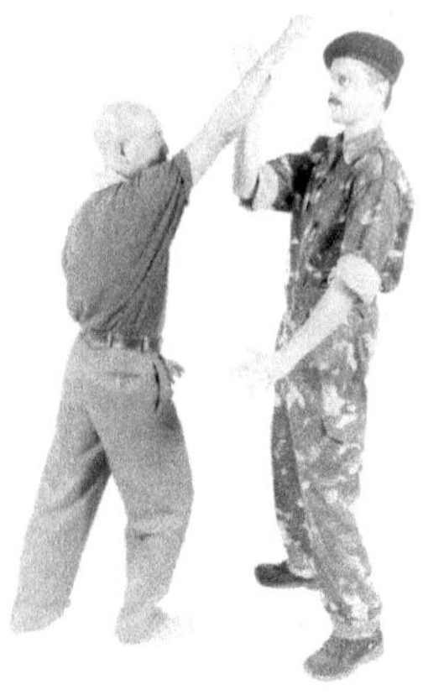

1. Your opponent tries to grab your hair with his leading hand (right hand). Stand in a steady stance, with body weight divided equally on both the feet, position your hands to react for any attack. As soon as the opponent strikes, block with the outside block with your right hand.

2. Step forward with the left foot and hold the opponent's wrist with your right hand and bring it to at the waist level. Simultaneously lift your left hand above the opponent's hand, as though you are ready to pin his hand under your left arm.

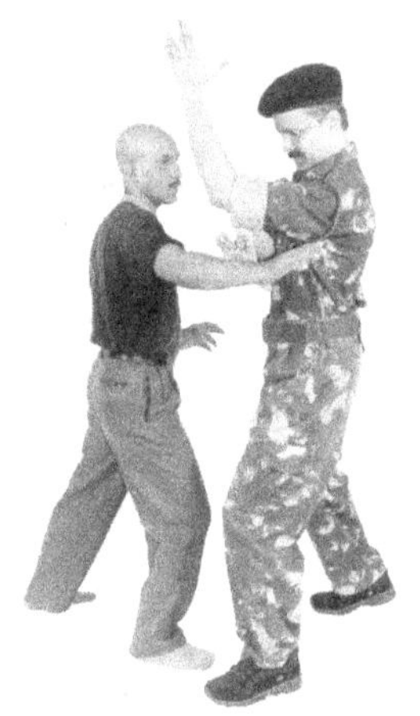

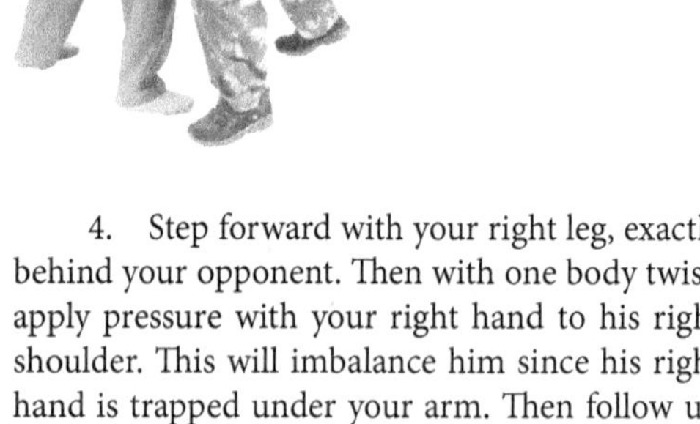

3. Pin your opponent's right hand under your left arm, twist your whole body weight to your left leg and feign to strike with your right hand.

4. Step forward with your right leg, exactly behind your opponent. Then with one body twist, apply pressure with your right hand to his right shoulder. This will imbalance him since his right hand is trapped under your arm. Then follow up with any counter attack techniques.

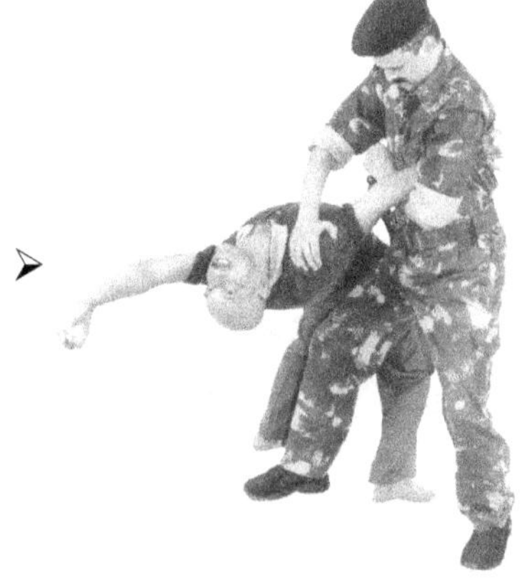

Techniques 11:

1. The attacker is armed with a knife, and is
ready to lunge it into your abdominal region, you
are supposed to check his advances, with your eye
movement on his knife without provoking him. Pull
in your abdomen region if the knife comes near your
body and keep your hands in on guard position,
ready to defend yourself.

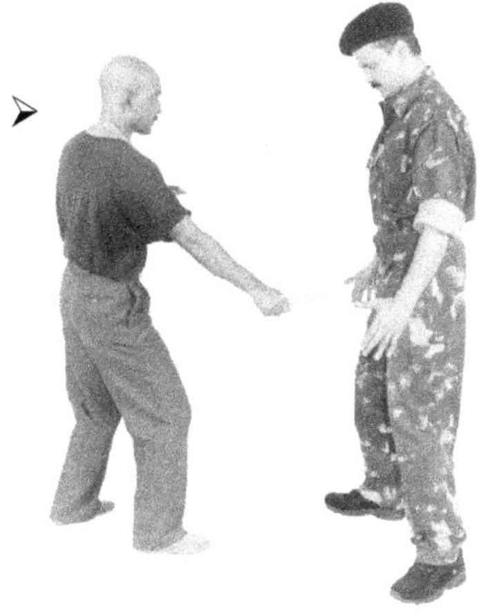

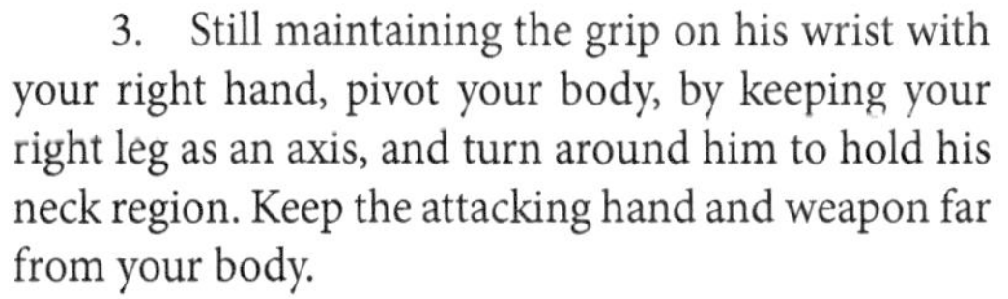

2. Step with your right leg to his extreme
right and simultaneously hold the wrist of his right
attacking hand, with your right hand. Your left
hand is on guard position.

3. Still maintaining the grip on his wrist with
your right hand, pivot your body, by keeping your
right leg as an axis, and turn around him to hold his
neck region. Keep the attacking hand and weapon far
from your body.

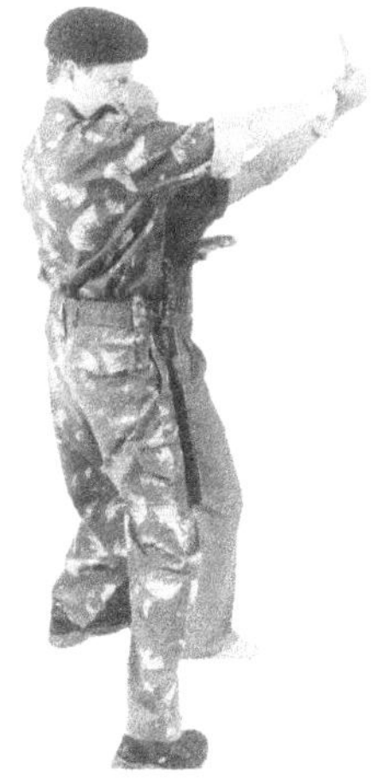

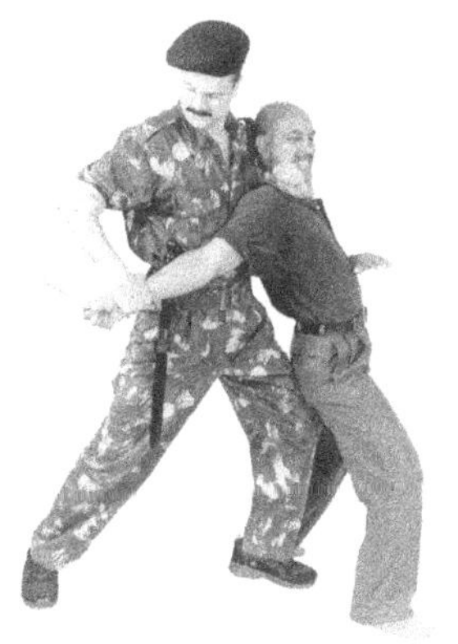

4. Immediately side step with your right leg
towards your extreme left and pull his right hand
towards your waist and lock his elbow on to your
hip, this will give him intense pain, since his elbow
is locked and neck is choked, and then follow up
with any counter attack techniques.

Techniques 12:

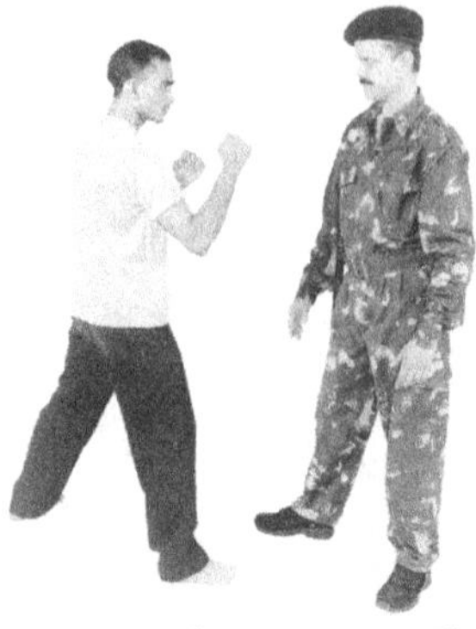

1. Your opponent's is on the verge of throwing a punch with his leading hand to your face level, you are supposed to check his advances, with your eye movement on him without provoking him. Keep your body weight evenly on both the legs and be ready with your hands in on guard position, ready to defend yourself.

2. The moment he starts his attack, immediately take a side step with your left leg to his right side, trap his attacking hand with your left hand, with the right hand hold his opposite side shoulder, so that he does not slip away.

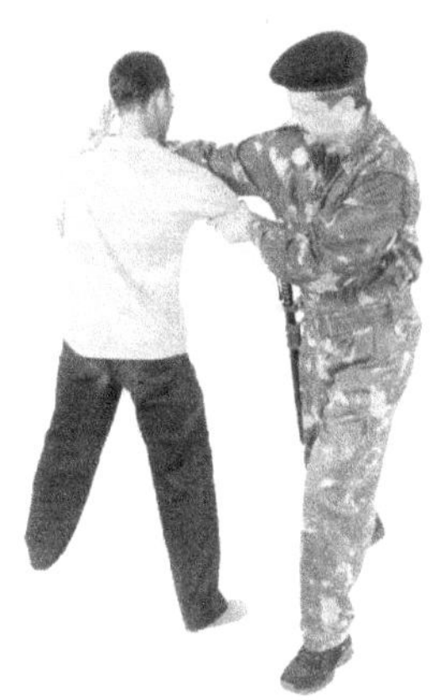

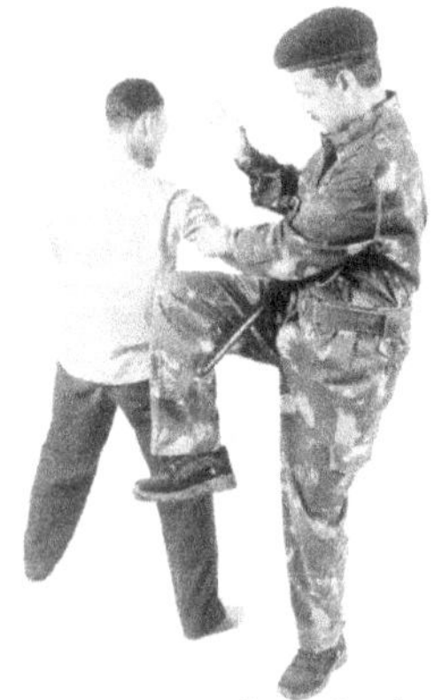

3. Now lift your right leg ready to kick the back of his knee, and pull his right hand towards you.

4. Kick the back of his knee with your right leg and immediately punch his right ear with your right fist, this will create tremendous pain and he will loose balance.

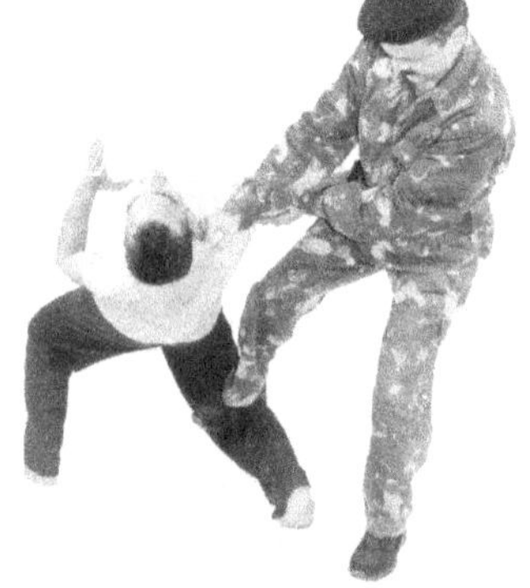

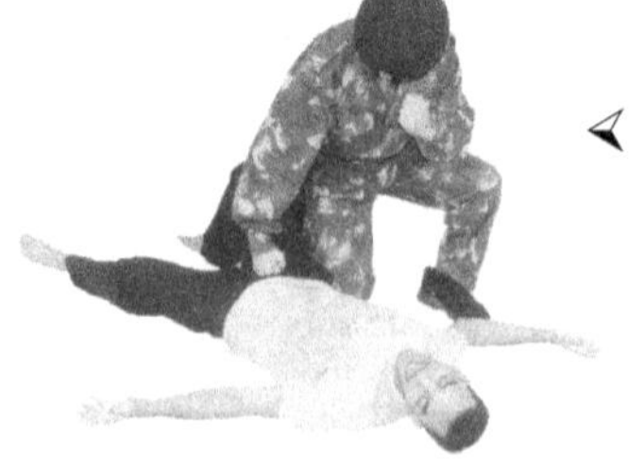

5. Then swing your body towards the left side, and hold his collar with your right hand and pull him down. With this movement he will loose balance and fall down, then with your right fist strike his groin region, with this strike he will be totally cold.

Techniques 13:

1.   The attacker charges in front and holds 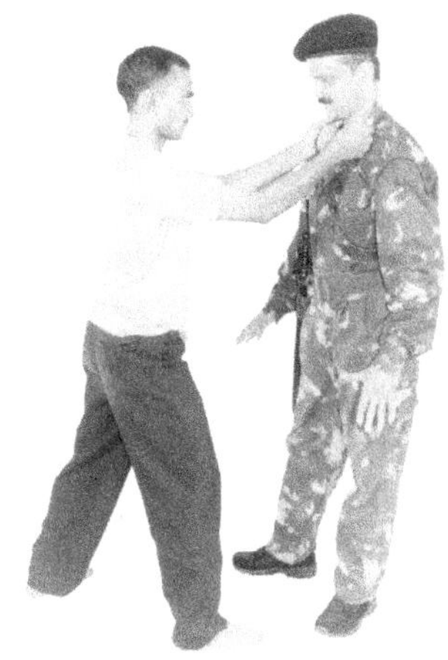 your collar with both his hand in a very threatening manner. Be steady and maintain your balance on both feet. Also check his advances, by keeping an eye over him without provoking him. Keep your hands in on guard position, ready to defend yourself.

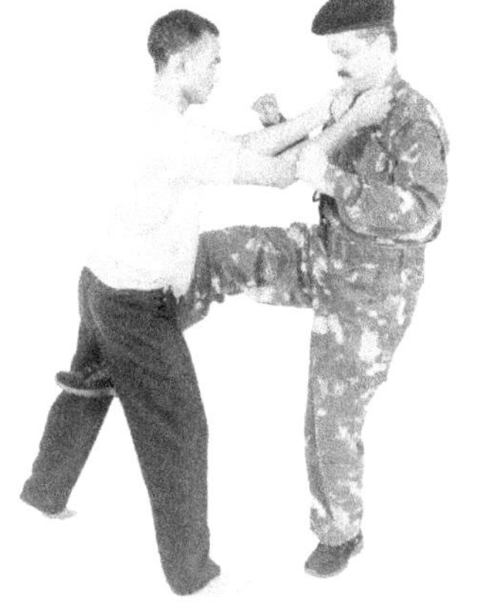

2.   Transfer your body weight on your left leg and lift your right leg to kick the opponent's groin, simultaneously press both your hand on his forearms.

3.   Hold both his elbows with both your 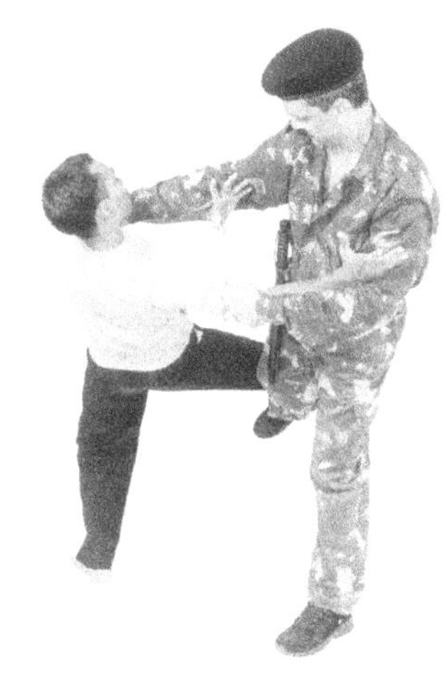 hands and recoil your right leg and kick your opponent's right leg, with your right leg towards his right ankle, and simultaneously swing your body towards the left, this will create an imbalance in the opponent.

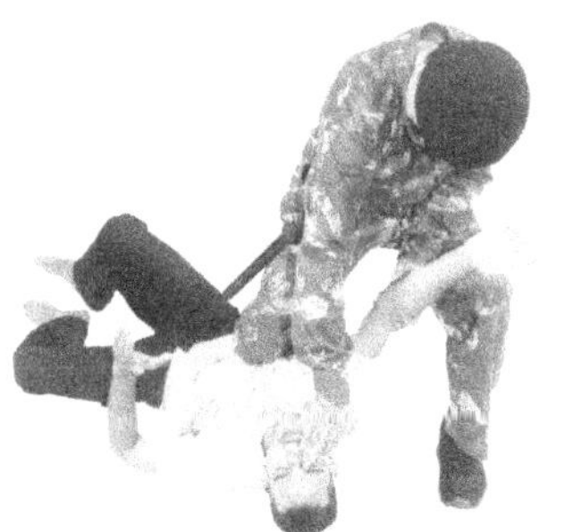

4.   Continue the swing till your opponent is pinned towards the ground, then immediately strike with your right knee towards his abdomen region, and then do a finger stab to his eye, this can blind him. **Use this technique only when all life saving methods fails.**

Techniques 14:

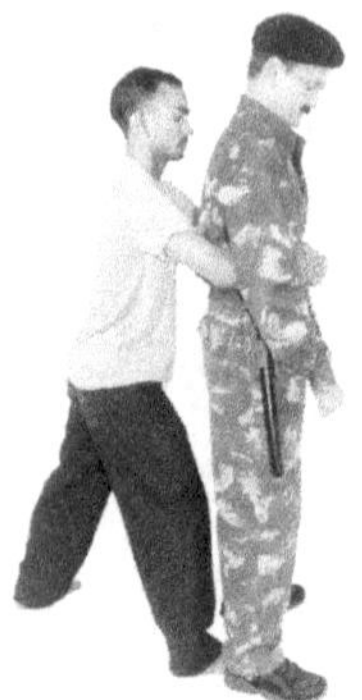

1. The attacker charges in and holds your waist from behind with both his hand in a very threatening manner. Be steady and maintain your balance on both your feet. Also check his advances, by keeping an eye over him without provoking him. Keep your hands in on guard position, ready to defend yourself.

2. Slightly shift your body weight on your left leg and swing around and bang your right elbows to his jaw line, this will weaken his grip.

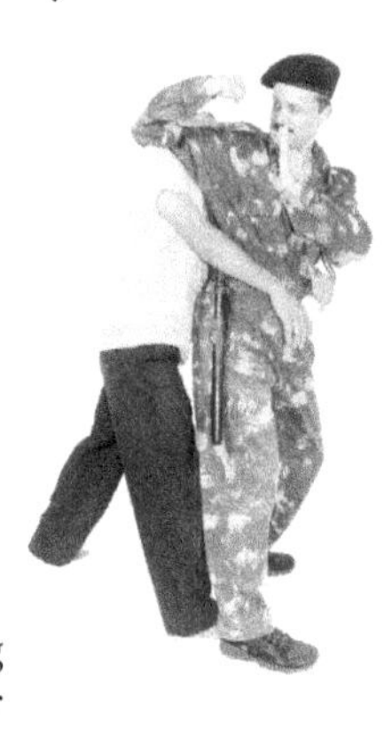

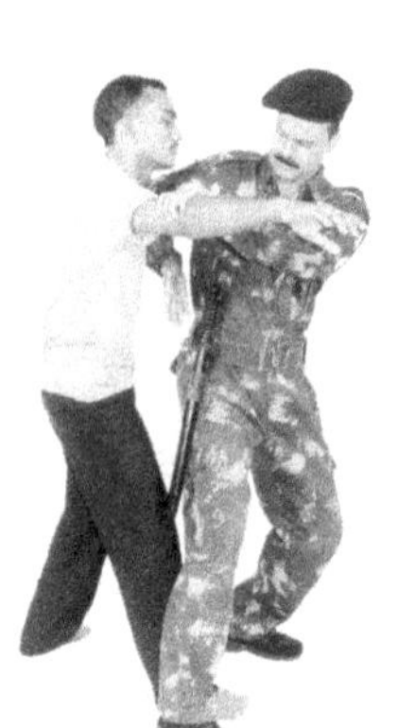

3. Slightly slip your right leg a little to your right and take your right hand in between you and the opponent, as though you are about to hold his waist from the other end. Hold his right hand with your left hand.

4. Hold your opponent's waist and lift him up on your hip and swing his body towards your left side, by transferring your body weight from right leg to left leg. Maintain the grip on his right hand with your left hand, so the throw can be successful.

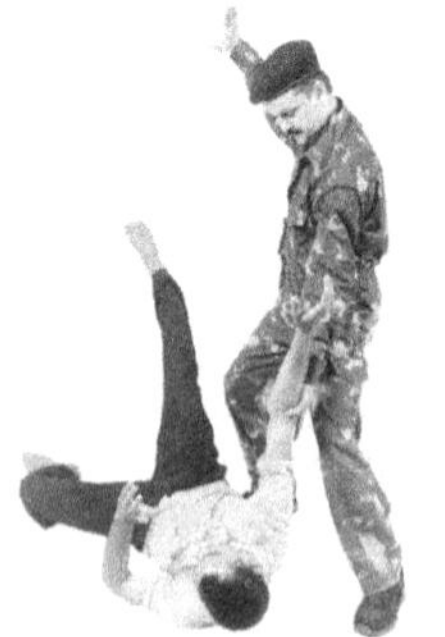

5. When the opponent is thrown completely on the floor, follow up with any counter attack technique, so that it will discourage him for any future endeavor.

Techniques 15:

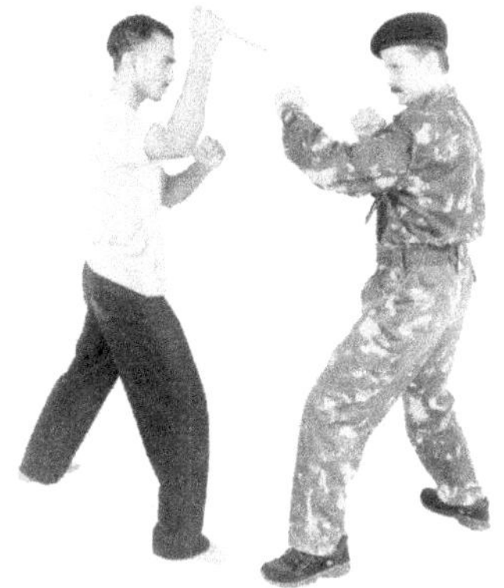

1. The attacker is armed with a knife, and is ready to lunge it into your chest region, you are supposed to check his advances, with your eye movement on his knife without provoking him. Keep your hands in on guard position, ready to defend yourself.

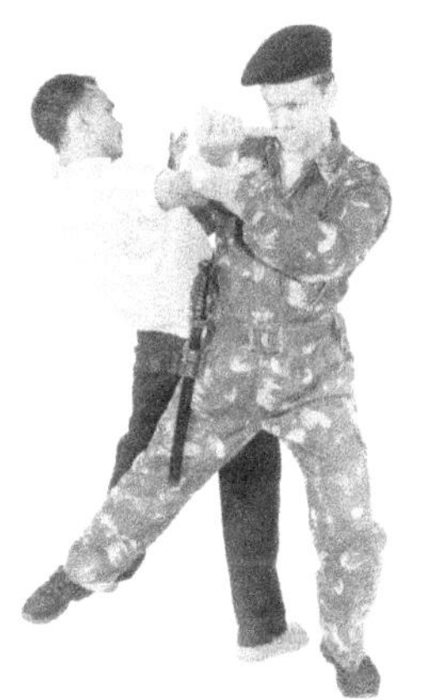

2. Finding a good opportunity slip your right foot behind him, and hold his attacking hand with your left hand and slip your right hand around his wrist and hold your left wrist with your right hand, this will imbalance him.

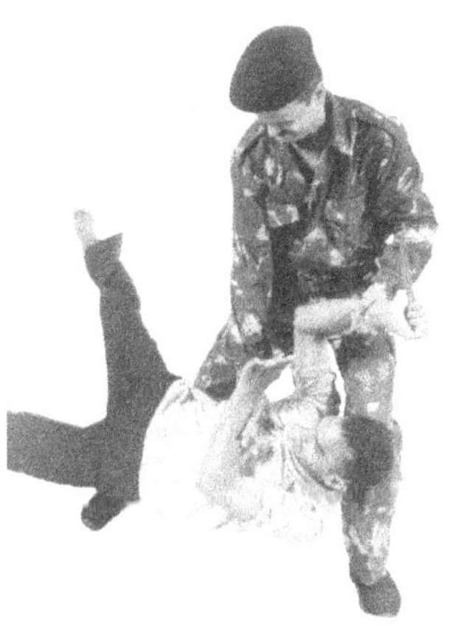

3. Immediately turn your waist towards your extreme left and swing the gripped hand in the same direction, you will find your opponent flung on the floor, and then you can counter him with any of the attacking techniques.

Techniques 16:

1.   Your opponent's is on the verge of throwing a chop to your neck region with his leading hand. Immediately try to control his attack with your leading hand (left hand) and simultaneously with your rear hand (right hand) try to trap his other hand. Your body weight is on the leading leg.

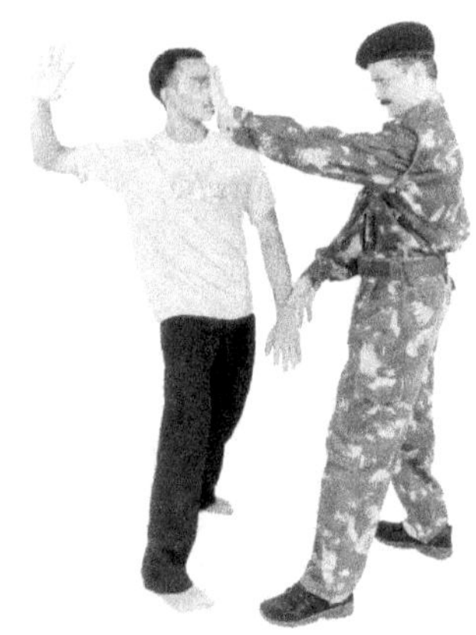

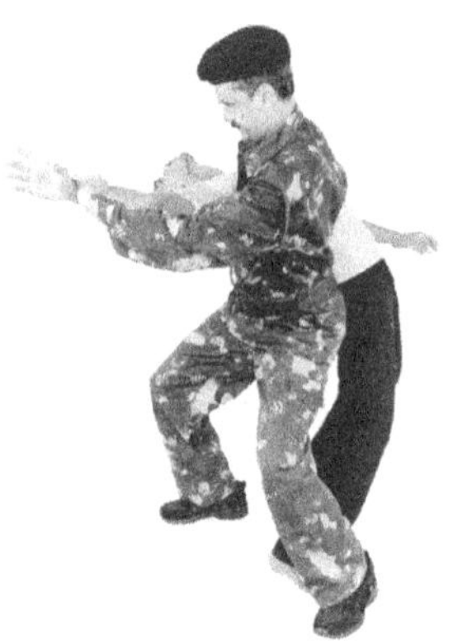

2.   Simultaneously step with your right leg behind his right foot, and hold his leading hand (right hand) with your left hand. Without loosing any time, hold his waist with your right hand. Body weight equally divided on both the legs.

3.   Gripping his waist tight, swing your body towards your extreme left side by transferring the body weight on your left side. Pull the opponent's right hand with the flow of the movement; the opponent will be totally airborne.

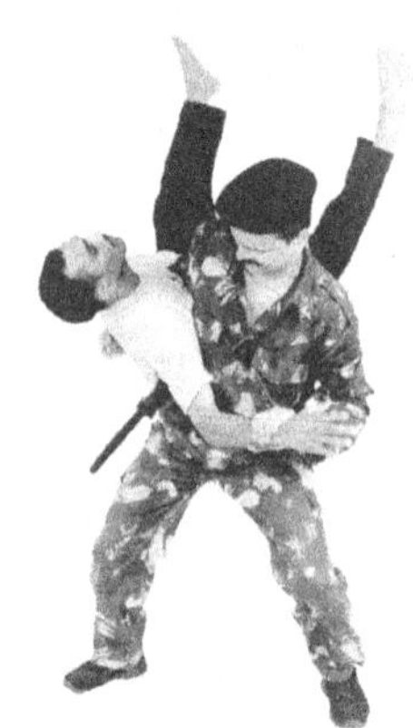

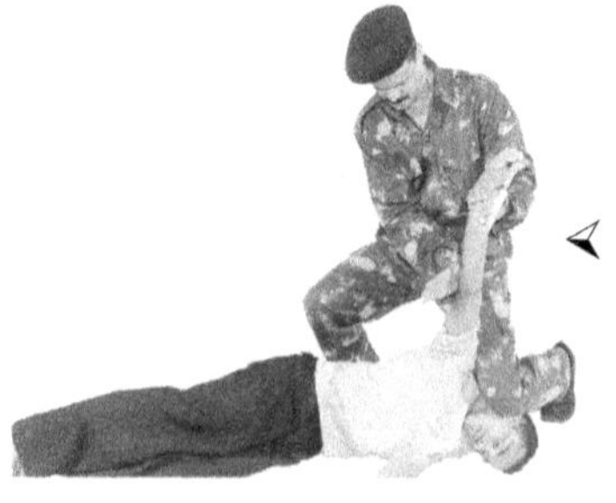

4.   When your opponent is totally flung down on the ground, then follow up with any attacking techniques.

As a student of Self Defense, do not commit the mistake of ignoring techniques based on

- *BITING*
- *CLAWING*
- *GRABBING*
- *PINCHING*
- *HAIR PULLING*
- *FINGER BREAKING*
- *SPITTING*
- *HEAD BUTTING, etc.*

Usually these techniques work best in close fighting, but with practice they can be made to work very effectively in long distance fighting also.

❑   ❑   ❑

This page intentionally left blank

Chapter 8

Armed Techniques

There is no deadlier weapon than the Will!
The sharpest sword is not equal to it.
Use your weapons with prudence, only when the situation demands.
Use your creativity as the first means of preventing DANGER.

Armed Techniques

Although the art of weaponry had enjoyed a glorious past its future remains doubtful. Modern culture leads people away from the study of ancient weapons for a variety of reasons. First, guns with their ease of operation and greater killing potential have made people believe that understanding martial weapon is impractical. Secondly, very few qualified masters are around to teach and thereby preserve the artistry of handling ancient weapons. Finally, becoming proficient in any weapons requires much time, patience and practice. In today's society, few people appear willing to exert the energy necessary for learning the ancient art of weaponry.

Martial art weapons tend to be outlawed immediately on exposure in the media. Either law is passed naming them as illegal, or existing laws are interpreted to include them. So the next best weapon is the **STICK**. Many a times a civilian may not be able to avail the facility of a stick. Sometimes it becomes very cumbersome to carry a stick only for self defense purpose. The next best weapon, which can be found in day to day life are umbrella, walking-stick, hockey stick, broom, water-pipes, pen, belt, etc. which are just another derivative of the stick, and can be found anywhere. Selection of the weapons from the above mentioned materials depend on the site of the incident, how easily it is available and how well versed you are in that weapon.

Warning: *Complexity of the situation and the severity of life saving can force one to take lethal weapons; otherwise please do not indulge in such practices. Since each and every life is precious, they do contribute something or the other to nature and society. Never act in anger, be cool, calm, think and then react.*

Points to be noted against armed attacker:

1.   An armed attacker has a huge advantage which must not be underestimated.

2.   Great care must be taken that you do not provoke the use of the weapon.

3.   Show no resistance at all.

4.   Talk and look for opportunities to act.

5.   Deal with the weapon before the man.

6.   Move out of the line of attack as you act.

7.   He may try to confuse you by flicking his knife from one hand to the other, if he is   an experienced fighter, and then avoid him like a plague.

In case of multiple attackers:

1.   Always attack the leader of the pack, which may help the others to change their   minds.

2.   While defending, constantly keep on changing position by zigzagging, ducking,   spinning and weaving.

3.   Try to crash the attackers into each others.

4.   At any cost don't trip or fall on the ground.

5.   Position yourself, where you can handle them one at a time, play total safe.

Situation 1:

1)   Your attacker looks like a desperado, who has decided to harm you with the sword, square in front of him by keeping an eye on the weapon.

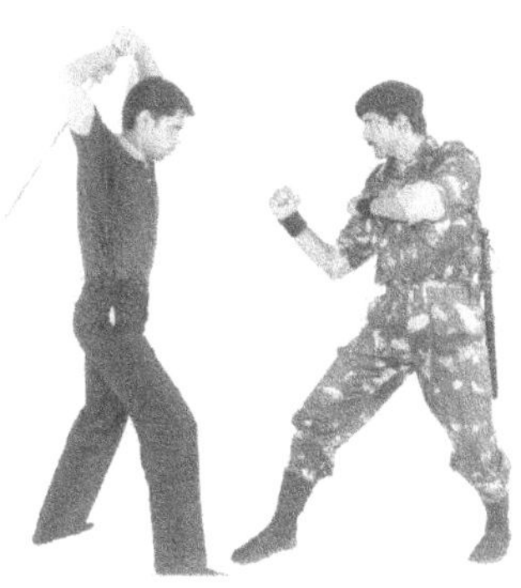

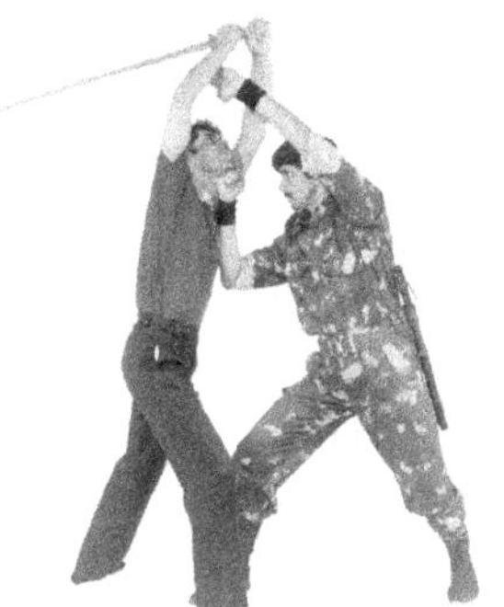

2)   The moment he lunges on you step with your leading leg and simultaneously deliver a hook punch to his jaw, simultaneously the other hand guarding or controlling the opponent's weapon.

3)   Immediately duck your body and slip your leading hand under his groin to hold his leading leg, simultaneously your rear hand will hold the weapon hand of the opponent, the whole movement looks like you are just about to uproot his balance.

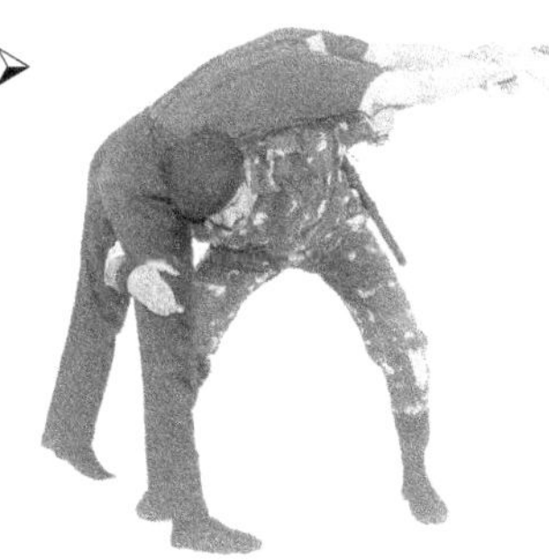

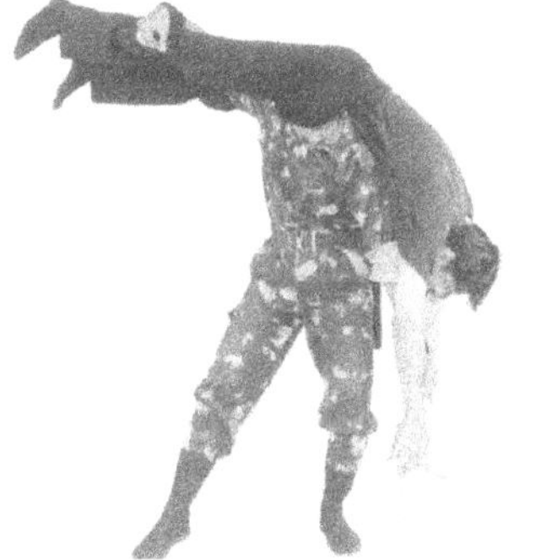

4)   Continue the motion of lifting and throwing your opponent over your shoulder, note that he lands on his head. All the above movement has to be executed in one smooth motion. Practice hard, one requires a little strength to execute this techniques.

Situation 2:

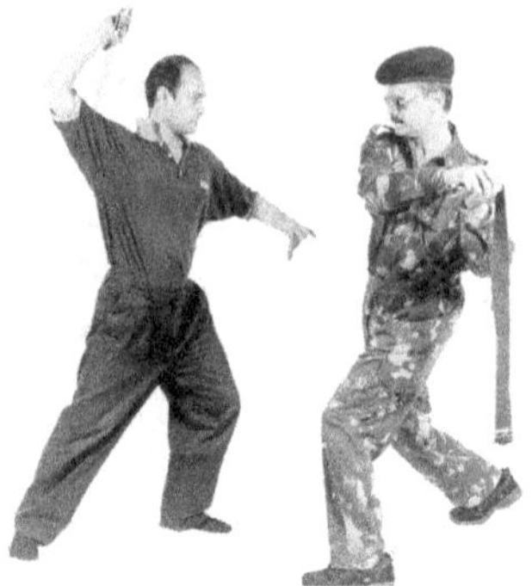

1. Your attacker is ready to attack you with a chopper, with his rear hand; simultaneously you should be ready with your belt or any flexible weapon to smash into his face, by keeping an eye on his weapon.

2. The moment he lunges on you, turn your waist by transferring your body weight on the rear leg and swing the belt on his neck region.

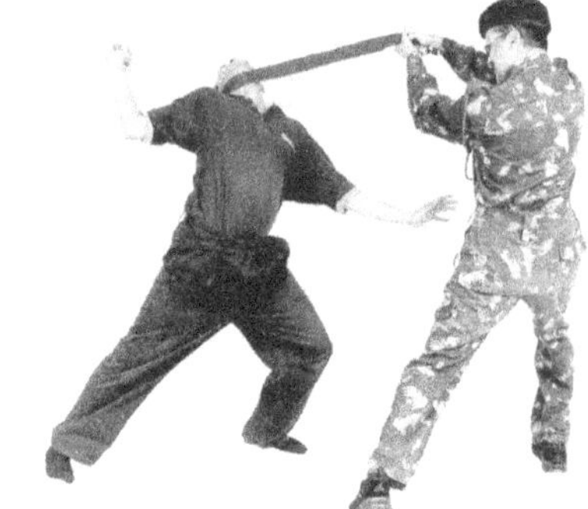

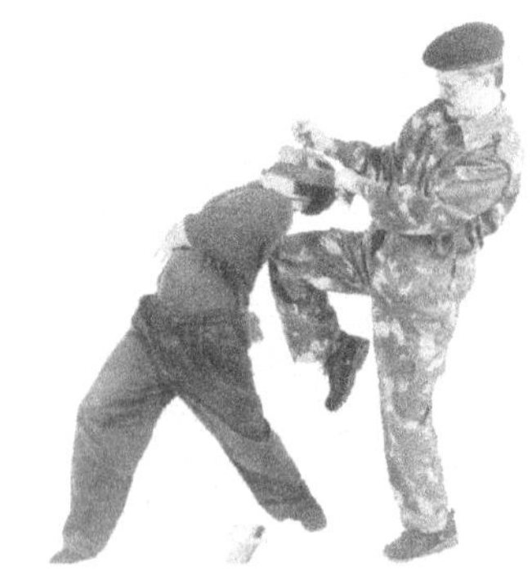

3. Automatically the belt will coil around the opponent's neck, make use of this motion, by immediately holding the other end of the belt, and choking his neck with the belt. This move will create confusion in the opponent's move and his grip on the chopper will weaken down.

4. Immediately strike with your rear knee into his kidney region, this will weaken his balance and automatically, he will fall down and he will be at your mercy. All the above movement has to be executed in one smooth motion. Practice hard, one requires a little skill and dexterity in the movement to execute this techniques.

Situation 3:

1. Your attacker is ready to attack you with the chopper, with his leading hand; simultaneously you should be ready with your hands on the belt, by keeping an eye on his weapon.

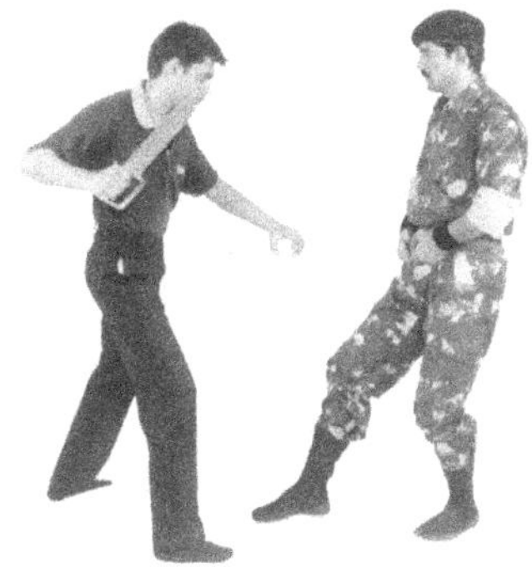

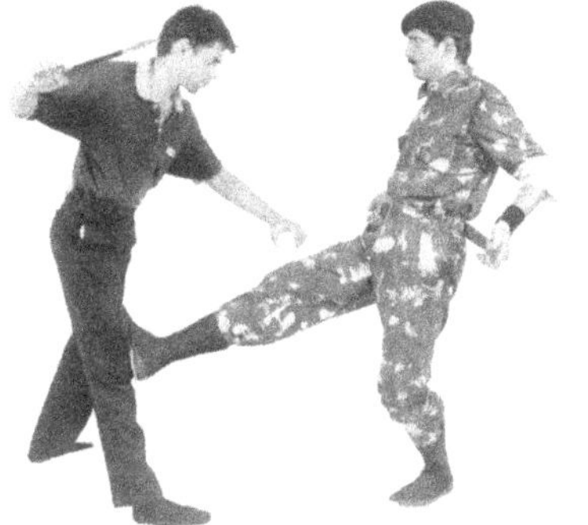

2. The moment he tries to make any move, kick his leading leg knee, by your leading leg, this will jam his movement and will give him partial paralysis in his leg region, simultaneously unloosen your belt.

3. Immediately remove the belt from behind and above your head, to bang it on to his neck region, since the kick has made a mark on the knee region, hence your opponent is in pain and he is bending in front.

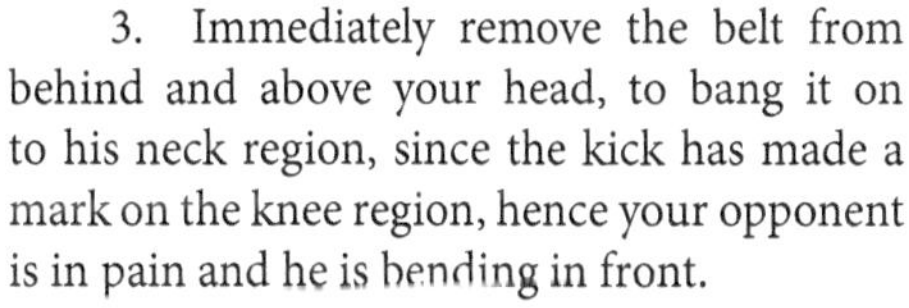

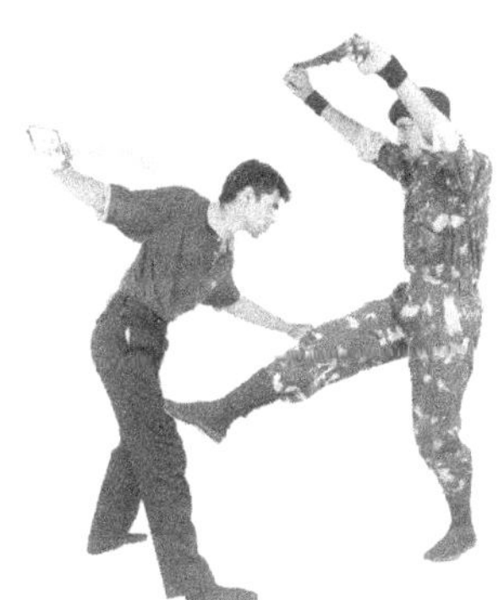

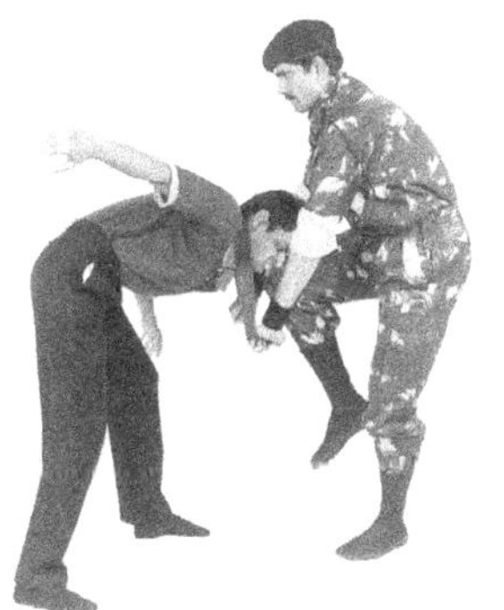

4. Without loosing any time, pull the belt on top of his neck and down, simultaneously pull your leading leg slightly behind and thrust your knee straight on to his nose, this will give him a bloody bruise, and the grip on the chopper will immediately weaken down. All the above movement has to be executed in one smooth motion. Practice hard, till one achieves fluidity and dexterity in the movement to execute this technique.

Situation 4: Attacked while fallen down.

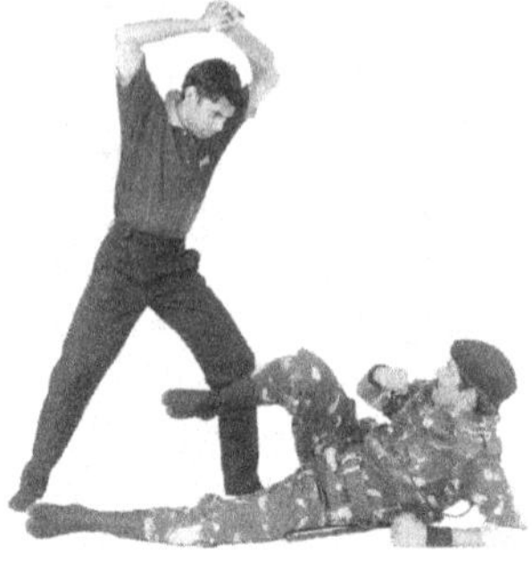

1.   It may happen that you will be knocked to the ground. This is a very dangerous situation for you and it may be a very bleak chance that you may be in such position, but still better to be prepared, than to surrender. When the attacker pounces on you with his sword, take proper support of your body with the help of your hand, and be ready to jam his attacking range, with your leading leg, eyes on the weapon.

2.   The moment he moves in kick his groin, with your leading leg, keeping your leading hand in on guard position.

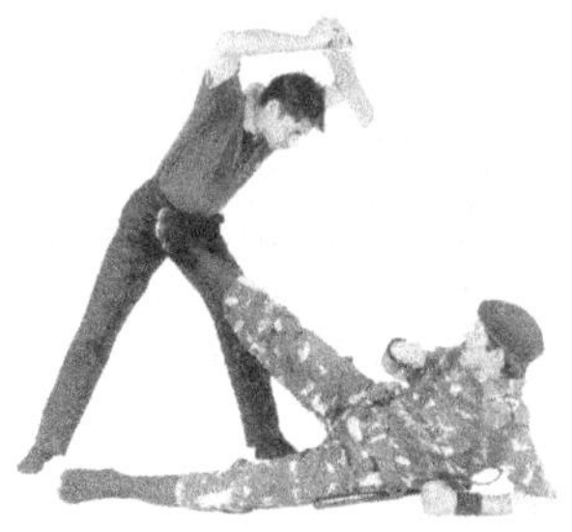

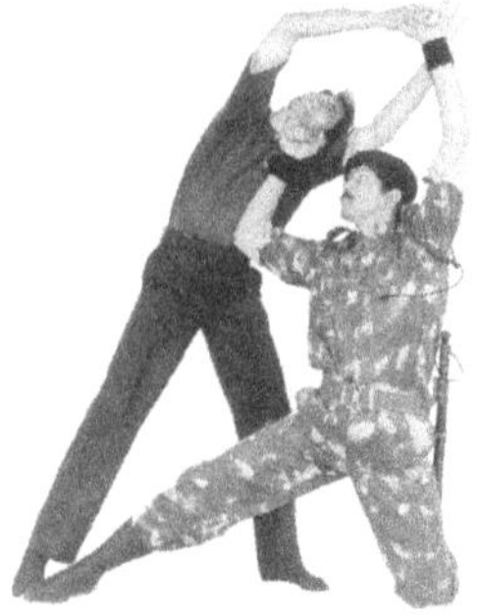

3.   Immediately place the leading leg near his rear leg and spring up like a cat by bending the rear leg and placing the body weight on this kneeling leg, and simultaneously double up with a hook punch to his jaw region, while the rear hand will hold the opponent's weapon hand, This will shake him up, and he will loose control over himself.

4.   Immediately choke his neck with a strong vice like grip, and push the shoulder of your leading hand into his chest, then drag him over and across your shoulder as shown in accompanying figure.Remember while doing this movement, your rear hand will be on the weapon hand, and this same hand of yours will act as a fulcrum to throw him across your body.

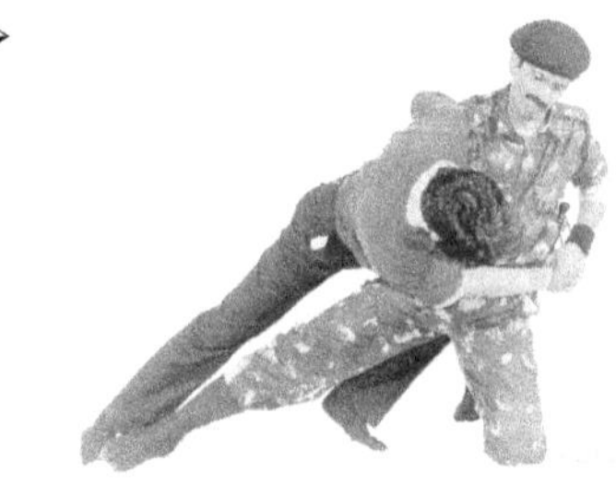

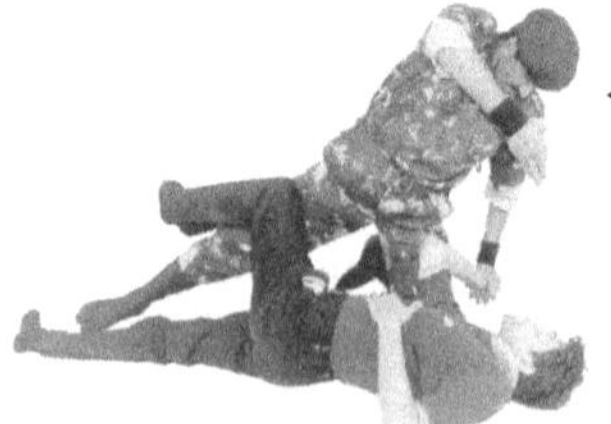

5.   Immediately, after throwing him down, pounce on his body like a tiger to deliver a finger stab either to his eyes, side of neck or to the hollow of his throat. All the above movement has to be executed in one smooth motion.

❑   ❑   ❑

Appendix I

There are many types of unarmed fighting styles which emphasize the development of power as their main objective. In fact it is not necessary to know how much power, or how much conditioning has to be done to hit a specific point, so that some damage could be incurred on the opponent. But any blow which is landed with sufficient force to any specific point will be effective. The fallacy of this method is that it will not work for small people. A man of 45 kgs. would have great difficulty developing enough power to hit indiscriminately against a 80 kgs. adversary.

The other argument against 'power theory' of unarmed fighting is that it assumes constant, continuous training, which is not a practical idea. Finally women and children cannot hope to learn a form of self defense which depends on power development. To make self defense effective and practical with only normal or moderate strength, one can set the target within the four line of the body and learn how to deliver effective blows.

• **Target Setting:** To deliver an effective blow or a damaging one to any vulnerable point, one should set the target at least six inches behind the point of contact (or above or below the point of contact for specific points). E.g. if the point of contact is at the nose, then set the target at the back of head. All strikes and kicks should have enough power to set the damage, but always remember do not sacrifices speed for power.

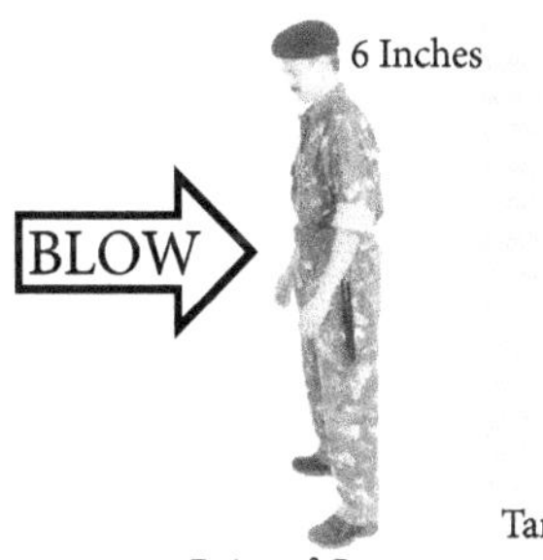

• **Concept of four lines of the Body:** To deliver an effective technique one should always remember the four lines of the body. From the neck to head region is called high line. From navel to neck region is called middle line. From knee to navel region is called low line and from sole of feet to knee is called lower low line. Any blow coming to a particular region, it should be blocked or dodged in that particular region, without wasting energy and time, (for more details see Chapter 3 of Basic Defensive Move). If you see an opening in any region, strike at that moment very swiftly, without wasting time, energy and balance using the technique from Chapter 5 of Basic Attack, also remember to set the target effectively.

FOUR LINES OF THE BODY

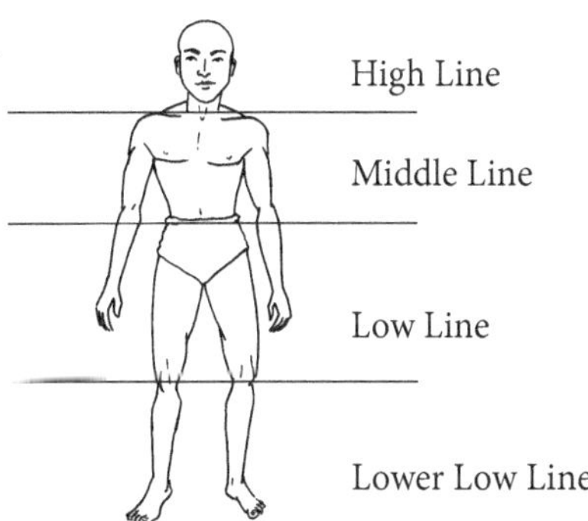

-        **36 Vulnerable Parts of the Body:** To make self defense effective and practical with only normal or moderate strength, to the most vulnerable areas of the opponent's body one should practice hitting the vulnerable points accurately. While practicing, care should be taken especially of points which are very sensitive, for they can be damaged with minimum power, so that your partner does not get injured. A blow to any of the underline and bold print points could be fatal or lead to a very serious and irreparable injury.

12 Back Points:

1.   **<u>Base of Skull</u>**

2.   Below the ear lobe

3.   **<u>Seventh Vertebrae</u>**

4.   Between shoulder blade

5.   Vertebral column

6.   Back of upper arm

7.   **<u>Under last rib</u>**

8.   **<u>Kidney</u>**

9.   Tail Bone (Coccyx)

10.   Back of thigh

11.   Back of Knee

12.   Achilles tendon

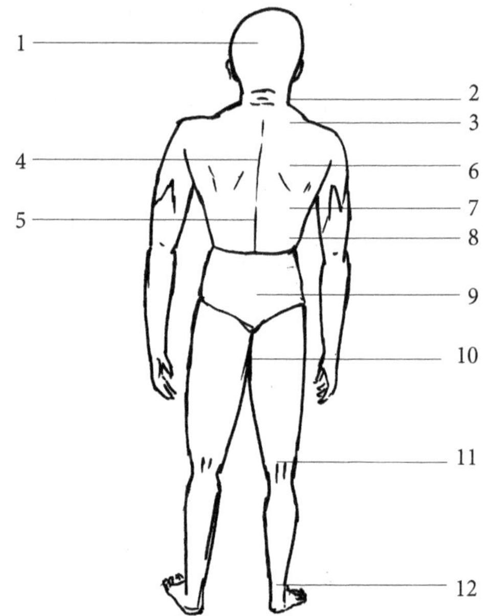

24 Front points:

1.   Hair

2.   **<u>Temple</u>**

3.   **<u>Eyes</u>**

4.   Nose

5.   Jaw Hinge

6.   **<u>Ears</u>**

7.   Under the jaw

8.   **<u>Windpipe</u>**

9.   **<u>Hollow of throat</u>**

10.   Collar Bone

11.   **<u>Chest (Breast Bone)</u>**

12.   **<u>Solar Plexus</u>**

13.   Arm pit

14.   Inside of arm

15.   Forearm mound

16.   Rib cage

17.   Last rib

18.   **<u>Stomach</u>**

19.   Navel

20.   **<u>Bladder</u>**

21.   **<u>Groin</u>**

22.   Inside of thigh

23.   Shin Bone

24.   Instep

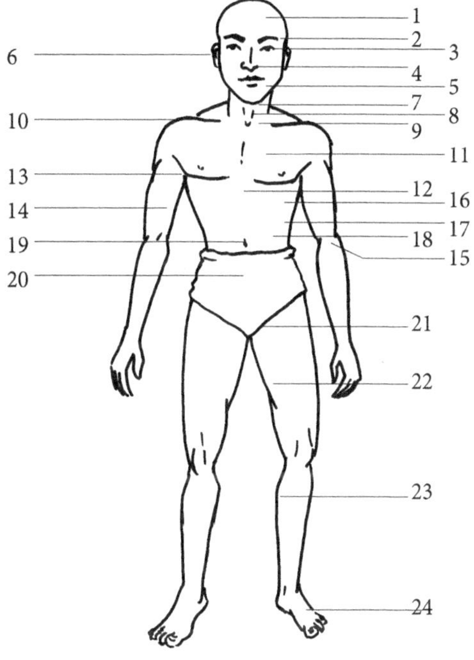

Appendix II

Your attacker reads your body language long before you begin your defense. Typically in self defense training, we focus on specific fighting skills. Body usage, or how you hold and maneuver your body, contributes to your ability to perform a specific skill such as a kick, parry, joint lock, etc., but often we forget how fundamental our body usage is to the effectiveness of the technique. In general how we hold and use our body influences potential attackers whether they are on a training floor, in the street, working with us as business associates or simply friends and family. As a result, our body signals and the psychology behind them become extraordinarily important. Both researchers (psychologists, sociologists, etc.) as well as martial arts masters have written about body usage. It can be very instructive to compare the information and learn from it.

Certainly Gichin Funakoshi, founder of Shotokan karate, understood the importance of body usage. The mind and body, he said, should be trained and developed in a spirit of "humility" which is a somewhat old fashioned term for respect and unpretentiousness. In fact, it is in the fundamental aspects of self defense such as standing position (natural stance), moving position (the transition between stances), and orientation to others that body usage is most important. Let's begin by examining the natural stance to discover the implications and significance of body usage to both the martial arts training floor and the "real world".

From a psychological point of view, the natural or ready stance is an opportunity to practice projecting power or authority in order to control a potentially threatening situation. Police officers, for example, are trained to exude an image of authority in order to control criminals, an un-victim like; confident and vigilant demeanor position is required in order to discourage attackers from selecting you. For power in the workplace, one should note that "authority is as much nonverbal as verbal." The basic authority stance which is almost "military in nature: the shoulders squared, the head erect, the jaw muscles tight, the mouth closed and unsmiling, feet planted firmly on the floor and eyes steady." As you can see, the ready stance has similar dimensions for martial arts, business, military/police, and practical street defense. For a better understanding of why and how the ready stance works, let's look at some of the specifics.

Eyes to front (not down or averted): Police reports confirm that a potential attacker will often "test" you through eye contact. If you show submissiveness by looking down or to the side, you may find yourself mugged. Likewise, criminals have told researchers that they prefer to attack people who are looking down. This is such a common attribute of mugging victims that psychologists have labeled it the "downcast demeanor". Keeping your eyes forward is a sign of attention and intent. If a person acts distracted, with behavior such as brooding, staring at the sidewalk, searching through a purse or bag, or reading a map, are found to be more likely to be attacked. Another cue that assailants seem to notice is head and eye movement. People with exaggerated or furtive eye movements or sweeping side-to-side head movements - which may imply fear, preoccupation, or being off guard - are more likely to be assaulted.

Chin in (so the head is not tilting back): The goal here is to keep the neck relatively straight and upright. The head, which weighs about 3-5 Kgs, is a wonderful self defense tool and can be used to strike forward or backwards. For optimum balance and comfort to the neck, however, Alexander Technique teachers recommend allowing the head to be "poised lightly on top of the spine". The common saying, "it's a pain in the neck" illustrates how easy it is to create discomfort here. Alexander Technique is a body usage training system that teaches people how to move in the most natural and easy manner. It also unlocks the flow of physical, mental, and spiritual energy to higher levels of well-being and effectiveness. Alexander Technique training is much in demand by people in the performing arts (including martial artists) and is frequently prescribed by medical specialists to relieve pain that other treatments have not been able to address. One of the guiding concepts of Alexander Technique is to mentally repeat to yourself the following body usage mantra: Let the neck be free, to let the head go forward and up, to let the back lengthen and widen. Letting the chin drop allows the top of the head to lift upward and the neck to move freely. Royalty and successful warriors returning to their home cities are often described as entering with "head held high". Thus the chin/neck/head position conveys stature and maintains your health.

Shoulders lowered slightly in a natural posture (not raised, not slouched, and not hunched): Often we raise our shoulders to shrug (a sign of uncertainty or disinterest) or to indicate surprise. Tension in the shoulders will also cause them to appear raised. All of these attributes - tension, surprise, uncertainty, and disinterest - illustrate un-readiness which translates into vulnerability. By following the Alexander Technique, guidance of neck free, head forward and up to let the back lengthen and widen, the shoulders will find their natural, lowered position without turning inward in an ugly, unhealthy, hunched shape. Typically in upper middle class homes, children are taught to sit and stand up straight because that is correct and appropriate behavior. Slouching or slumping are habits associated with lower status or position in life. Indeed, we call someone a "slouch" when we want to imply that they are awkward, lazy or inept. Likewise, a slumping or hunched posture is associated with low energy, poor body coordination, and low self-esteem. In martial arts, having your shoulders lowered but upright presents an image of confident ability.

Lower abdomen flexed slightly: The goal here is to avoid arching the lower back, but rather to let it release into length. Height is a natural deterrent to aggressors. Supporting this concept, research at the University of Helsinki, Finland, found that taller women conveyed more authority. Although you can't increase your height, standing with a straight posture can give you a taller appearance. When you have an erect, or an upper-middle-class body posture, other people, regardless of their background, find you more attractive, intelligent and competent - all of which are likely to deter an attacker both on the training floor and in real life. Another goal of flexing the belly muscles is to create a sensation and attitude of readiness. Like a spring, a slight tension as opposed to total relaxation of belly muscles prepares the martial artist for action. This activity is as much mental as physical since any manifestation of tension will be interpreted as weakness and will impede action. Body connection is another martial arts way of phrasing the desired result to be achieved by flexing the lower abdomen. Again, both mind and body are involved to create a consciousness of total effectiveness and the appearance of effortlessness.

Legs straight without being locked at the knees: As with flexing the lower abdomen, an important body usage aspect here is the avoidance of tension. Too much tension in the muscles around the knees constricts blood circulation which can cause you to be light headed or even to faint, a situation that has embarrassed some men at their own wedding. Hence keep knees slightly bend when standing for long periods.

Right foot about a half step from the left and toes pointed outward slightly: For good body usage, the placement of the feet should always optimize balance. In a standing position, this means that each foot should be under the corresponding shoulder which, as Funakoshi directs, is approximately a half step apart. Turning the feet outward a little achieves a slightly broader base, further improving balance. From a self defense point of view, you should keep your body motion to a minimum. This means you should consciously stand still rather than shifting your weight from one foot to the other. Shifting your weight can be interpreted as uncertainty, a sign of vulnerability.

The fists about two inches in front of the upper thighs, fingers toward the thighs: Keeping your hands free and in front of your body conveys readiness on your part because it is clear that you can use your arms and hands to block or strike if necessary. In addition, you should keep your hands and arms close to your body because large gestures can be misinterpreted as insults. Likewise, avoid crossing your arms or shoving your hands into your pockets as these may be considered threatening behavior. The great Okinawan karate Master Gichin Funakoshi is quoted, "that one should stand calmly, ready to react to any circumstance". Wherever we are, combining our knowledge of body usage with Funakoshi's instructions will allow our standing position to de-escalate potential problems in the real world.

Kiai: There is a tradition in the Oriental martial arts of using the voice as a weapon. This is known as the kiai shout. It is said that a strong kiai can stun an attacker or knock birds off trees! If you don't believe, then go and listen to a lion roar at the zoo and you will perhaps understand. The shout is used in two ways. Firstly it is roared straight at a, would be attacker to stop him in his tracks, and secondly it is used in combination with the various defense moves. For example, when used with a punch it is roared out as you make the move. This not only affects the attacker but concentrates the power in the defender's body and in the defensive move. The shout itself must originate from the lower abdomen, i.e. three inches below the navel. It must be extremely loud and forceful and be an expression of one's whole body and of total fearlessness.

❑   ❑   ❑

Glossary

Aikido	:	a Japanese art of controlling the opponent move, with his own energy, thus becoming one with the opponent's movements in order to control him/her.
Baithaks	:	squats.
Chi kung/Qigong	:	science of controlling breath, a biophysical energy is generated through breathing techniques, which is most popular in China.
Judo	:	the Japanese art of self defense employing mostly of throwing and strangulation techniques.
Karate	:	a Japanese art of unarmed combat, also called the art of empty hands, which employs all parts of human anatomy to punch, strike, kick or block.
Ninja	:	A Japanese warrior hired as spies, and assassins, in feudal Japan.
Shotokan karate	:	a Japanese art of unarmed combat, it is characterized by powerful linear techniques and deep strong stances.
Wrestling	:	science of grappling.
Yoga	:	science of harmonizing body and mind, developed in India.

Bibliography

1. The Art of Kung – Fu Wu – Shu : by Christopher Fernandes,
   (Chinese Martial Arts) Zorba Publishers, 1996.

2. The Art of Stick Fighting : by Christopher Fernandes,
   (A Comprehensive Self Study Guide) Zorba Publishers, 1998.

3. Self Defense : by Syd Hoare,
   Hodder and Stoughton, 1982.

About the Authors

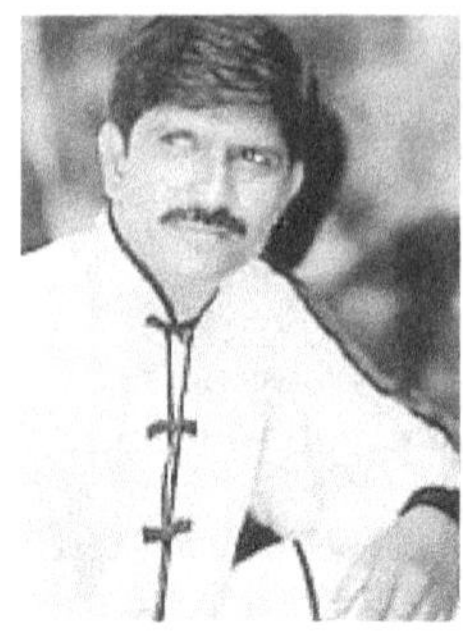

Mr. Christopher Fernandes born in 1962 was trained in "Hua – Chuan Kung – Fu" by the late Lama Sevang Migyuar Nobu. Mr. Christopher Fernandes became the first Indian to be trained in Beijing, China. In Beijing, he was trained in the seven competitive routines. Lui Xian Dong world No.1 practitioner for Drunken Sword also trained him. He completed his "Chi Kung or Qigong" training under Dr. Rong Yi Qun. In 1993 he was the official observer for the Second World Wu-Shu Meet at Kuala Lumpur in Malayasia. In 1994 he was instrumental in conducting the first Wu-Shu Judges seminar in Orissa for "Wu-Shu Association of India". He choreographs martial arts sequences for Commercial Ads, TV serials, films and simultaneously coached many of the film stars in Chinese Martial Arts. His earlier three books, "The Art of Kung Fu Wu Shu, The Art of Stick Fighting, and Tai Chi Chuan" were a great success.

Mr. Lazarus Mascarenhas born in 1959 was trained in "Hua – Chuan Kung – Fu" by the late Lama Sevang Migyuar Nobu. He was the first teacher to teach Chinese Martial Arts in the suburbs of Kalyan and Thane. In 1988 he founded the UMARC in Mumbai. He has conducted various workshops and seminars on Martial Arts and Holistic Fitness, based on Oriental Breathing technique. Mr. Mascarenhas was also the editor of UMARC's news bulletin. He was also instrumental in conducting the first District and State level Chinese Martial Arts Tournament at Andheri, Mumbai in 1989 and 1991 respectively. Since the last few years he has trained scores of students including security personnel, in Armed and Unarmed Combat.

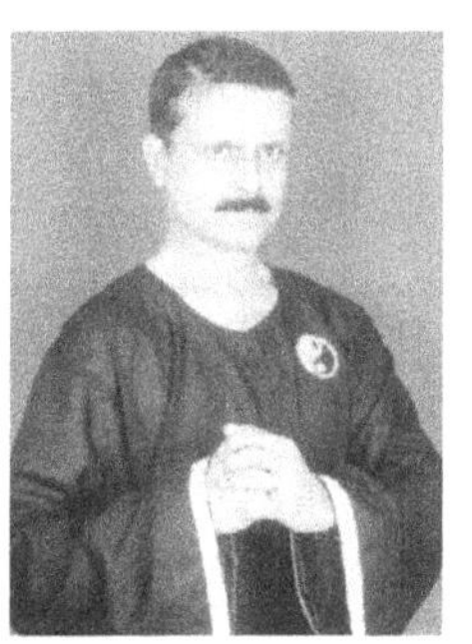

❑   ❑   ❑

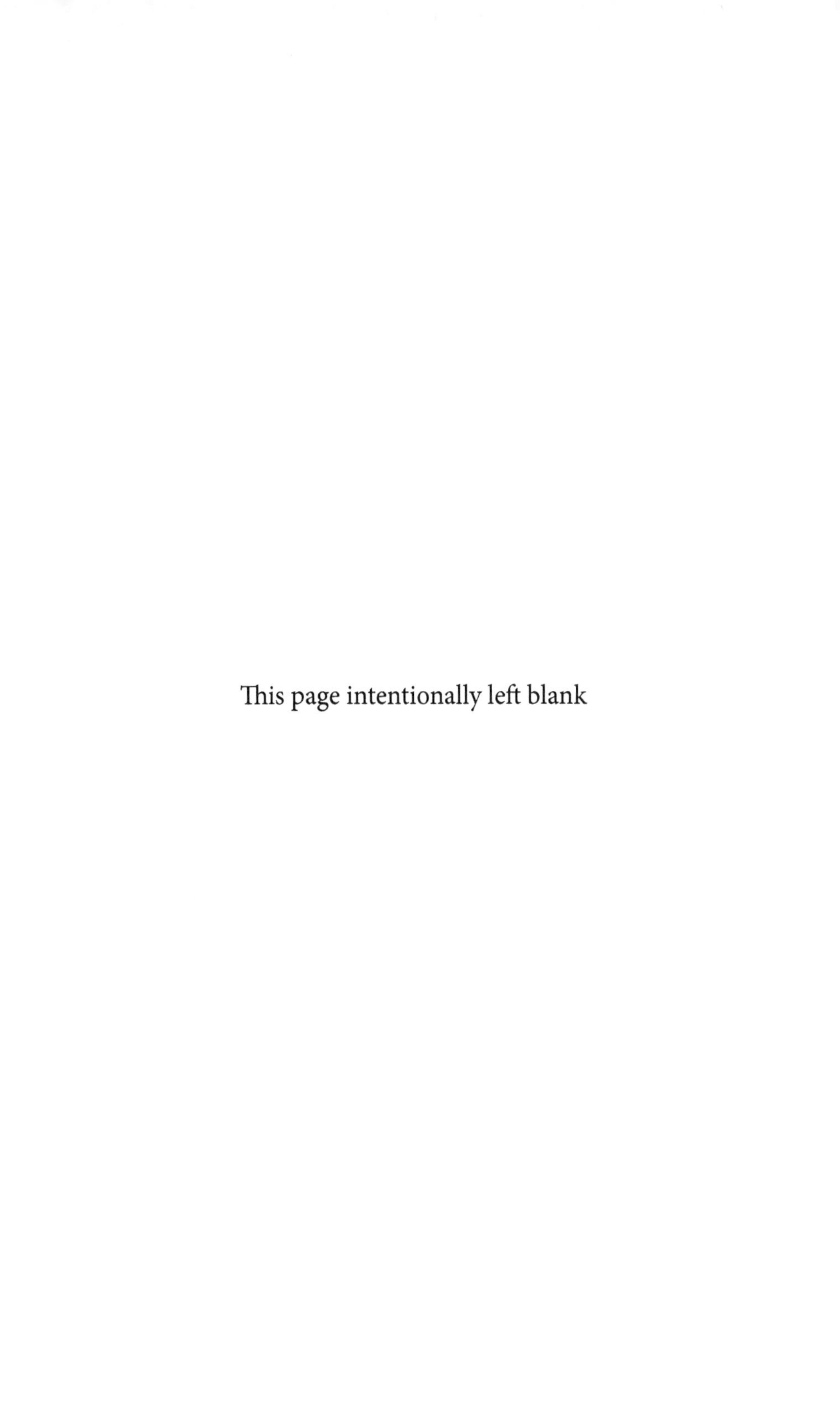

This page intentionally left blank

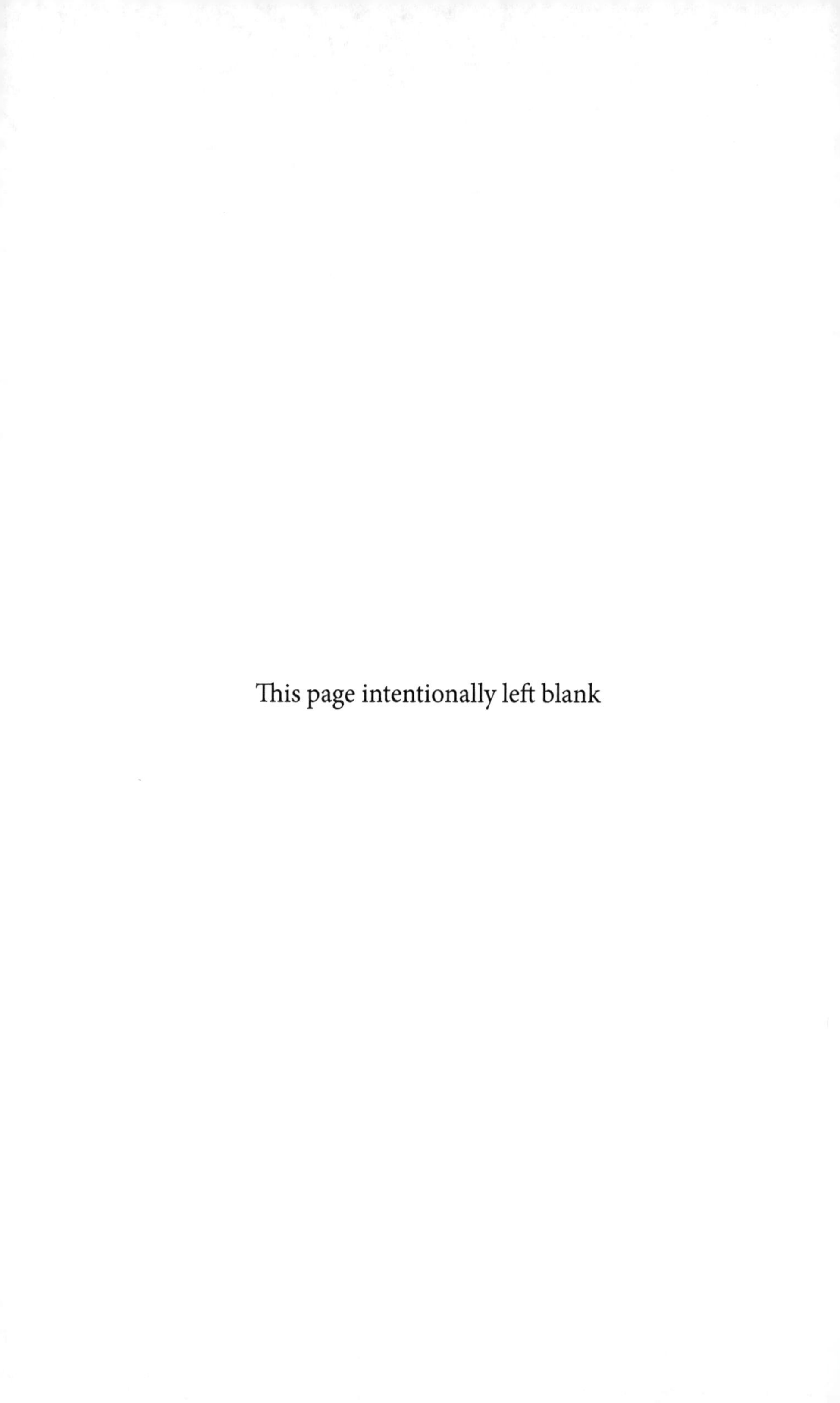

This page intentionally left blank